Jabs, Jenner

and Juggernauts

A Look at Vaccination

By

Jennifer Craig, Ph.D.

II

Cover Design by Presto DesignWorks

ISBN 978-0- 9559177-4-5

Website: www.fearoftheinvisible.com

**Published by Impact Investigative Media Productions
Leonid, Bristol Marina,
Hanover Place, Bristol, BS1 6UH.
U.K.
Tel. (44) (0)117 925 6818
Cell (44) (0)7970 253931
Email   jan@janineroberts.com**

Impact was founded in 1985 in Australia, where it produced award-winning films and books on the colonization of Aboriginal lands. Since moving to the UK in 1990, it has produced investigative films seen on the BBC, WGBH (US and Canada), ABC (Australia), Channel 4 in the UK, as well as investigative books and articles on blood diamonds, public heath, biology, spirituality, environmental and human rights issues.

Cataloguing Information for this Work.

Health: Vaccination
History: Public Health
Ethics: Medical
Indexed.

Dedicated to the memory of

Dr. Charles Creighton, 1847–1927

Acknowledgements

No book is written without help and encouragement and I have many people to thank for the production of this book:

Verna Relkoff, my long-time teacher, for editing so ably and for all her useful comments.

Nicola Harwood for the creative non-fiction class where I started this.

My invaluable writing group: Anne de Grace, Susan Andrews Grace, Joyce MacDonald, and Rita Moir for consistent encouragement and painstaking critiques.

Viera Scheibner, Hilary Butler, Edda West, Sheri Nakken and Janine Roberts for checking the manuscript for accuracy. Janine also for finally seeing the book through to publication. Special thanks to Hilary for the title.

CONTENTS.

Preface

It is a privilege to know Jennifer Craig, nurse, grandmother, PhD and author; a woman who, after a lifetime working for the public health system in hospitals and medical schools, has, in the great tradition of Florence Nightingale, dared to challenge the medical establishment. She now calls into question the science behind giving our new-borne infants more and more vaccinations in order to "protect them" from epidemics that in the West were mostly defeated, not by vaccines, but earlier with the provision of clean water, sanitation and good food.

In this book written with clarity and humour she takes us back to little-known early days of vaccination, revealing a history that has led us into disasters; a history today buried and rarely mentioned, especially by the pharmaceutical 'experts' who promote their drugs as if they, not the hygiene movement, defeated the Victorian epidemics.

She shows how the foolish arrogance of the early days of vaccine research has been translated today into a "medical evangelism' where vaccine science is taught as if a religious doctrine that it is forbidden to doubt.

She goes into the legal consequences for parents and explains the salesmanship that underlies the recent vaccines such as that against cervical cancer or HPV. She describes how vaccines are contaminated during the very process of manufacturing, leaving them littered with parts of dead cells, mutagenic DNA fragments and multiple viruses from different species, all these never mentioned in the official lists of 'vaccine ingredients.' It is like giving a recipe for 'cake' and never mentioning that the ingredients are mixed with sewage.

She tells how the polio vaccine has long been dangerously contaminated with monkey viruses, including one implicated in many human cancers. She includes devastating statistics – devastating that is to those who maintain that vaccines stopped epidemics – and reveals, as only a nurse can, how diseases really are defeated.

She describes the myths that sustain a multi-billion dollar industry – and the idleness of journalists who do not question. She begs parents to investigate the risks involved in vaccinating their children and the need for this. If there is any doubt, the precautionary principle should rule. Don't do it unless you are sure.

If we cannot learn from history we are condemned to repeat it.

There are fundamental questions that need to be asked in my view. Key among these is how accurately are viruses identified and proved to be the only cause of a diseases, Do uninfected cells also make them? Could viruses be sometimes the result of a disease, not the cause?

We also need to know how viruses are produced for vaccines and how sanitary is this process? In scientific circles, this is no great secret, but it is rare for it to be explained to parents – and this is no great surprise when one discovers just how it is done.

Take for example the measles virus. How is it produced for measles vaccines? How pure is this process? There are official instructions provided for doing this by the leading US government agency that monitors epidemics and researches viruses., -- the Centres for Disease Control (CDC). The instructions it gives to medical technicians are currently, as I write, up on its website. 1[1] Their title is "Isolation and Identification of Measles virus in Culture."

It instructs: first obtain from a patient with spots, and other clinical symptoms of measles, a small sample of fluid, say saliva from the mouth or some urine. Put this in the fridge. Presumably the measles virus sought is in it – but no need to look for it now.

Next you have to prepare in the laboratory a cell culture in which this virus will hopefully multiply so you have enough to use for vaccines and for research.

How to do this. The CDC instructs: first obtain a marmoset monkey. It recommends this species as it says its cells are '10,000 times' more sensitive to the measles virus than are normal human cells, meaning they are much more likely to fall gravely ill during this procedure. Now when cells are removed from a living being and placed in a laboratory culture, they will start to mutate as they struggle to survive. This factor is commonly ignored by the medical technician or pharmaceutical company – but it too can lead to unpredicted consequences. (In order to save money, the measles and MMR vaccine manufacturers are currently using cells from mashed chicken embryos for the final mass production phase.)

Now, states the CDC, extract cells from the monkey. Commonly this is done by removing its kidneys and testicles, and mashing them as these organs are the easiest for an amateur surgeon to locate.

The monkey cells are then settled into a one-cell-deep layer in a laboratory vessel. But they are not yet ready to be exposed to the fluid from the suspect human case of measles. First they have to be prepared.

First thing to do, the CDC instructs, is to 'immortalize' the monkey cells (done by exposure to radiation or toxins). In other words, you make them cancerous. But they are still not ready to exposure to the putative sample of measles virus. The next step, the CDC says, is to give them the dreadful Epstein-Barre disease!

After this, the very sick monkey or chicken cells are to be exposed to a poison. The CDC instructs: take care to use rubber gloves and splash goggles while adding to the cells a digestive toxin called trypsin.2[2] It warns to expect some of the cells to fall away as if they are poisoned. They have been. Trypsin starts to break them up for it is a digestive chemical. It is as if the cells have fallen into acid. The CDC then instructs: add nutrients and glucose and leave the

---

[1] CDC. *Isolation and Identification of Measles Virus in Culture,* Revised November 29, 2001.
[2] http://www.sciencelab.com/xMSDS-Trypsin-9927313

surviving monkey cells alone for two days. No need yet to look at them with a microscope.

The CDC now instructs; add to them the fluid sample from the patient; then, after an hour, inspect the monkey cells with a microscope to see if any have become distorted, or are floating free as they were after the trypsin was added.

If 50% or more of the cells are now distorted, the CDC claim that it must be the measles virus in the just added sample from the patient that caused these distortions, not the cancer, not the toxin! It has no doubts. It instructs; if 50% of the cells are distorted, 'scrape the cells into the medium' and then store the lot at 70^0C as an 'isolated measles-virus stock!'

For the CDC there is no need to verify the presence of the virus by looking for it. No need to check if the earlier poisoning and making cancerous may have caused these distortions. The medical technician is instead instructed to put the whole culture of diseased monkey cells, together with the toxin added, away in the fridge as an "isolate of the measles virus" and as a proof that the original child patient had measles!

What the measles vaccine manufacturers do when they receive the culture from the lab is filter off the vaccine from the diseased chicken cells they use, taking out particles larger than viruses but leaving in everything of the same size or less – before injecting into our children a noxious mess, including any chemicals they add.

MMR, and single dose measles vaccines, also contain bird cancer viruses – according to the World Health Organization. At a recent scientific gathering it reported that avian leukaemia virus is commonly present in measles vaccine (which they have only safety tested for 48 hours) and, the manufacturers admit, much chicken "cellular degradation debris' – bits of broken up chicken cells and scraps of potentially mutagenic DNA – remains in the MMR doses given to our children.[3]

A recent scientific paper disclosed: 'The presence of Avian Leukosis virus (ALV) in chick-cell-derived vaccines is not a new phenomenon; many instances of ALV contamination in yellow fever and measles vaccines have been documented.'

So what about other viruses? According to a Dr Dominic Dwyer. a leading virologist, what they do in the laboratory is to add a different toxin to a cell culture in order to persuade these very ill cells to produce a different virus such as 'flu.[4]

There is no virus that is not made by a cell. In biology some scientists see viruses as messenger particles that carry information encoded as DNA or RNA from cell to cell – providing cells with a vital information highway. At least 15% of our genome has been transported by viruses between cells. Maybe we should stop calling them viruses – as this word means a poison? They are like messages in bottles. In themselves they are totally inert. They have no survival

---

[3] See "Fear of the Invisible" by Janine Robert.
[4] *Ibid,* page 187

instinct. They cannot use the information they contain. They are simply containers of information that are a billion times smaller than the cells they serve, shorter even than a light wave.

Cells need to communicate. Evolutionary biologists have discovered that this sharing of information plays an absolutely vital part in our evolution – helping us stay safe. Many illnesses are due to this communication breaking down.

What our vaccine scientists have utilized is the cells' ability to produce different messenger particles when exposed to different toxins. What we still need to research is just why our cells do this and if these messenger particles sometimes trigger our immune systems?

Cells when sick of course could make poorly coded messages, and some messages might not be good for the recipients. Our cells can 'silence' the messages they do not want. It is not so simple as it once seemed . But this system of cells and viruses evolved to help cells remain healthy – and still does this. We live in an ocean of such particles. Plant, human, animal cells – they all constantly put much energy into making these messenger particles. We mostly live healthy lives while breathing them in all the time. It is as if they are the plankton in our ocean. We evolved to live with them.

We are thus part of a universal sharing of information. We are Gaia for the world within us. Nine out of ten of the cells within us are bacterial and serve us – as free-living cells that seemingly chose to live within us, to serve us and to help us remain healthy while giving themselves also a good life. Each of us is thus effectively a multi-racially community, a city made up by billions of such creatures, all of which are surprisingly intelligent in their decision-making. We remain healthy when the balance is preserved, both within us and in the world around us.

Janine Roberts   September 2009

Introduction

My father used to say, "Never believe everything you read in the papers." If he were alive today I expect he would add, "Nor watch on the television." But it is difficult to remain immune from the relentless propaganda sent out by big corporations and the governments which support them. I, for one, now wonder what the truth is behind everything I read or watch and ask myself, "Who stands to gain?"

The industry that particularly interests me is the giant pharmaceutical with its powerful "spin," a spin so strong it has threaded its way into history, legend, politics and religion. What began as a naïve, and somewhat disgusting experimental inoculation conducted by a less than qualified practitioner, Jenner, has become a cherished belief. We venerate the inventor, and a very profitable industry has grown by leaps and bounds around the development, production and sale of his 'snake oil,' a vaccine. I now fear that the injection of vaccines in the name of health may instead be destroying health.

For example, the incidence of autism in the USA, where all children, often by law, are vaccinated is now one in every 96 boys. In the UK in 2008 it was estimated to be one in 66.[5] Prior to 1970, autism incidence was 1:2000. Is there a correlation between autism rates and vaccination rates? Mention this possibility to most conventional Western, or 'allopathic' health practitioners and you may well be treated as though you had accused the pope of indecent exposure.

These are, however, the type of statistics that I gleaned as I began my foray into the murky world of vaccination literature; into its history, the pharmaceutical interests, the propaganda, the fear mongering that keeps people locked in belief, and the political interests that uphold the sacredness of the ritual of vaccination.

The topic of vaccination appears with amazing frequency in newspapers, magazines and the TV news. Invariably the spin is that vaccines "save lives" and prevent "deadly" diseases. After all, it was responsible for the disappearance of smallpox, wasn't it? For years I never questioned, or even thought about, the value of vaccines. I had my children and pets vaccinated without a second thought; it was the right thing to do. Then something happened, oh, about twenty years ago, that awakened my consciousness; just a little tweak at the time but enough to give me a

---

[5] http://bjp.rcpsych.org/cgi/content/abstract/194/6/500

"heads up" as they say today. Life moved on and vaccination certainly was not an engaging interest until I took a course in homeopathy.

My career had always been in allopathic medicine. I trained as a nurse in England and then emigrated to Canada when it was importing health care workers as fast as it could. In the seventies I became part of the phenomena of the "mature student." I studied with an intensity that I can only wonder at today. The result was a Baccalaureate degree in nursing, a Master's degree in education and a Doctorate in education. I then became an educational consultant, both in a medical school and in my own business where I served all the health professions.

I retired to Nelson, a small city in the mountainous Kootenay district of British Columbia. It is known for an alternative culture that includes chanting, smudging, dreadlocks and a variety of healing practices that range from classical Chinese Medicine to rebalancing. Throwing off my academic persona I entered wholeheartedly into this new world. I bought a felt jester's hat, called myself Madrone and set about the study of homeopathy. To some, these actions may be indicative of a severe mental disturbance – as indeed they were. But not, I hasten to say, a mental illness. I experienced a paradigm shift, if you will; a total re-examination of my beliefs about medicine and healing; a recalibration of my world view.

The homeopathy course demanded of me an essay on vaccination. This seemingly small assignment set me off on a reading path that, to date, has had no end. The more I read, the more questions come to mind. I became incensed as only someone can who has been hoodwinked for years and then discovers the truth. My family and friends grew tired of my tirades about my latest horrifying discovery so, instead of seething inside and giving myself a gastric ulcer, I decided to write a book.

There are many books on vaccination; some are quick reads for parents and others are academic reviews of medical literature. This book is about what I discovered from my readings. It is a personal account and a personal journey. It is not a scientific book – I have written enough academic articles in my life – but it is based on good science: verifiable statistics, accurate analysis and cogent synthesis. It includes anecdotes from my life and, in some instances, dramatic renderings of historical events that paved the way to our current perceptions about health, dramatic renderings that were often for my own entertainment and I hope for yours, the reader. For example, as I read about the life of Lady Mary Wortley Montagu, who introduced the idea of inoculation to the western world, it was easy to picture her in eighteenth century dress returning to London from Turkey, agog with excitement about her discovery of a cure for smallpox. I have written it as a stage scene but the dialogue is taken directly from her letters and writings.

This is not a dissertation about vaccination. The references I have used are not always from the original source, although many are. Some are quotations from other books. All the quoted statistics I use are verifiable and there is a list of references in the back. Furthermore, I have included what interests me about the topic rather than what may to others be the most important. Off-the-cuff remarks, howls of horror and incredulous exclamations have been ruthlessly removed by my editor. I was advised to "Let the readers feel their own anger or emotions."

Above all I want this book to be interesting. I hope it will encourage readers to ponder the questions that must and should arise about the practice of vaccination. In the larger picture, I hope it will prompt questions about the assumptions we hold dear about disease and health and that these will lead to the examination of, not only my references, but others.

More than anything I hope it encourages parents, every time they take a child for a vaccination, to insist — absolutely insist – that they are informed of the risks of such a practice and that they are fully aware that the vaccine is not a guarantee that the child will not succumb to the disease. If they are in any doubt whatsoever they should refuse to comply; they are, after all, guardians of their children as health authorities are not. In Canada and the UK, and in most civilized countries, vaccination is not mandatory despite the haughty dictates of some health professionals. Even in the United States where there is immense governmental pressure to vaccinate, there are exemptions.

Chapter 1

Awareness

A television set blocked the middle of the expansive window but my eyes were drawn to the scene outside. The purple sky, splattered with fronds of pink, rested on an unbroken range of white mountains. I thought a star had nestled on one peak until it began to flash and I realised that a plane was coming in to land at this northern British Columbia town.

"Beautiful view," I said to Jean, my hostess, who was busy in the kitchen behind me.

"Yes," she said as she came into the living room wiping her hands on a tea towel. "We love living here." She hesitated before saying, "Dinner's nearly ready but I hope you won't mind watching a local TV program. I don't usually ask guests to watch TV but it's about our public health unit. It will only be fifteen minutes."

At this time, I had a contract with Ministry of Health to develop a job orientation program for public health nurses in the province and was in town to seek advice from the local nurses. Jean had organized my visit and now she was treating me to dinner. She poured us each a glass of wine and we settled down to watch an interview with a father and the Medical Health Officer.

The father held a child, about 18 months old, in his arms. The child was limp: her neck unable to support her head. Her expression was vacant; saliva drooled from around her protruding tongue; unseeing eyes rolled from side to side; flaccid arms and legs jerked in an uncontrolled, aimless manner. Every now and again she uttered a short screech like some sort of exotic jungle bird.

A picture of a bright, laughing baby appeared in a superimposed frame. The child, Jackie, was dressed in a pink stretch suit and was reaching for a ring of coloured beads with an intent look on her face. Another picture: this time Jackie in her bath sucking a rubber duck. Then there were the grandparents proudly holding their first grandchild. They smiled at the camera as they supported their granddaughter with her feet on a table so she could bounce. All the time the pictures flashed by the current Jackie lay in her vegetative state, her peculiar cry interrupting the interview to remind us of her presence.

Jackie had been a normal, active child, the interviewer found out from the father, until she received her D.P.T. (Diphtheria, Pertussis and Tetanus) and polio vaccine. The parents, a conscientious couple, had waited until Jackie was eight months old (rather than the standard three months) to have the child vaccinated. A couple of hours after the shot, Jackie had begun to scream with the penetrating, high-pitched cry of the brain-damaged child. The 'cerebral cry' we used to call it in the sick infant's ward, a cry that indicates excruciating headache. For the next two days her temperature was 103 degrees. She continued to scream until the convulsions started. After about ten days the almost continual seizures stopped and Jackie became limp and unresponsive. She has been that way since.

The Medical Health Officer acknowledged that the vaccine was responsible. He was very sorry; these things happen sometimes. No, there's no way of predicting which child will have an adverse reaction. Yes, these reactions are rare; unfortunately some children must suffer for the good of all.

Conversation over dinner was subdued. We did not talk about the program and our discussion of my project lacked its former zest. I could not get the image of the damaged child out of my mind. Surely this was a one-in-a-million occurrence? Until then I had assumed that vaccinations did nothing but good; they prevented disease and saved people from death.

My earlier training as a nurse had instilled in me a sense of duty, a duty of care, a duty to the public we served. We embraced an ethic that our patients came first, that their health mattered and that we would do everything in our power to help them. The idea that something we did could cause damage shocked me. It was clear, even to the medically uninformed that Jackie had no future as a fully functioning human being. Her life had been ruined for the good of all? What? Since when has "collateral damage" become an acceptable part of public health practice?

My life moved on and the memory of Jackie became just that—a memory. Not until I studied homeopathy did she re-enter my consciousness. The course required a paper on vaccination and I began by listing questions to answer. How did the practice of vaccination begin? What does a vaccine contain? What is the evidence that the injection of this substance prevents disease? What are the side effects? I thought about Jackie. And how many children suffer from collateral damage?

Chapter 2

Lady Mary

The introduction of vaccines into the Western world began with Lady Mary Wortley Montagu (1689–1762), the daughter of the Marquess of Dorchester, a leading Whig politician. The Marquess maintained a hospitable table and Lady Mary as a teenager acted as hostess for her widowed father. As such she was expected to carve the huge meat joints of those days. Meat carving was considered an art requiring skill and strength and in order to master it, Lady Mary took lessons three times a week from a carving master.

Carving was not her only accomplishment; she became a well-known literary figure with published poems and essays to her credit. Alexander Pope was her friend for a few years, until an argument over an investment engaged them both in a flurry of abusive rhyming couplets in iambic pentameter.

I read Alexander Pope in my high school days, 'though not fondly. Miss Hardy, my English teacher, managed to suppress any interest I might have had in literature and it wasn't until I took English 12 in Canada that it was renewed. The pink textbook, *Adventures in English Literature*, that I still treasure, helped me see the progression of ideas in writing and its relationship to the social conditions of the times. Now I appreciate the satirical mockery of Pope's *The Rape of the Lock*, which had us, as schoolgirls, giggling. I didn't realise that Pope is responsible for such quotations as:

"A little learning is a dangerous thing."

"Hope springs eternal in the human breast."

Prior to their estrangement, Pope wrote a sympathetic poem for Lady Mary after she had smallpox in 1715. The disease left her scarred, with no eyelashes, and gave her the label of "the spoiled beauty." In higher circles, women who had suffered from smallpox used beeswax on their faces to cover up the pock marks. The problem was that standing too close to a fire melted the wax. To prevent this embarrassment, adjustable fire screens were strategically placed to shield ladies from the heat.[6]

Despite her disfigurement Lady Mary married Edward Wortley Montagu, a member of parliament, and they settled in London until he was appointed British Ambassador to Turkey in early 1717. The couple returned in 1718 when the following notice was posted in the court circular:

On the 3rd October, 1718.
Notice from Hampton Court
Mr. Wortley Montagu , being returned from his Embassy at the Ottoman Porte, this day waited on His Majesty.

Lady Mary resumed her place in London society. The following is a stage scene where Lady Montague greets a friend shortly after her return from Turkey: the dialogue is constructed from her writings.

*   *   *

The curtains open on a drawing room furnished in early Georgian style. Lady Mary, dressed in a pastel-coloured, full-skirted gown and a lace cap sits close to an Adam fireplace. A footman enters.

FOOTMAN: Mrs.   Griselda   Murray,   your Ladyship.

(The footman exits.*)*

LADY MARY: Griselda.   My   dear   friend.   How delightful to see you after all this time.

MRS. MURRAY Mary. Let me look at you. Are you much changed? No. You are well?"

LADY MARY   I am a little spent after our journey. I cannot tell you what discomforts we endured ... Hours in a carriage. You must know, I cannot sleep in a carriage. Then I was carried on the backs of porters over an Alpine pass. Such a prodigious prospect – mountains covered with eternal snow – but the cold, my dear, the cold. I still suffer. But come, my dear, come and sit by the fire and we shall take tea.

MRS. MURRAY You have a fine house here. And a prospect of the Piazza too. You will be able to see if Alexander approaches.

---

[6] Ransom, S. *Wake Up to Health in the 21st Century*. Credence Publications, 2003

LADY MARY   We were fortunate to acquire this house. Covent Garden is so delightfully central. And only 125 pounds a year.

MRS. MURRAY Shall you stay?

LADY MARY   I doubt for long. Edward will resume his seat but he may be called on another diplomatic mission.

MRS. MURRAY Shall you accompany him?

(Footman enters with tea tray, places it on small table and exits.)

LADY MARY   Of course. I long to visit the antiquities of the East. And that is where he will be sent, I suspect.

MRS. MURRAY I was greatly amused by your letters, But do tell me about the visit to the baths at Sophia that you made reference to.

LADY MARY   We were passing through Sophia and I wished to visit the famous hot baths. And there, in a marble-paved room, with cold fountains and steamy hot baths, were about 200 women in a state of nature, my dear, and I in a riding habit. Yet there was not the least wanton smile or immodest gesture. The lady that seemed the most considerable among them entreated me to sit by her and would fain have undressed me for the bath. I excused myself but I was at last forced to open my shirt and show them my stays.

(Lady Mary pours tea.)

LADY MARY   That satisfied them for they so believed I was locked up in a machine and that it was not in my power to open it! They attributed the contrivance to my husband. They thought that the husbands in England were much worse than in the East, for that they tied up their wives in little boxes of the shape of their bodies.

MRS. MURRAY And they so backward!

LADY MARY   Not in all things, my dear, not in all things. For I have brought home a useful invention that I will take pains to bring into fashion in England

MRS. MURRAY A useful invention, you say?

LADY MARY   Yes. A cure for smallpox!

MRS. MURRAY A cure for smallpox? That would indeed be a blessing. And, of course, having suffered that dread disease yourself ... Pray tell, how do they cure the smallpox?

LADY MARY   People send to one another to know if any of their family has a mind to have the smallpox; they make parties for this purpose. When they are met, an old woman comes with a nutshell of the matter of the best sort of smallpox and asks what veins you please to have opened.

MRS. MURRAY Oh no. I could not countenance it.

LADY MARY   Rest assured, my dear, the operation gives no pain. The old woman rips open the vein that you offer her with a large needle and puts into the vein as much venom as can lie upon the head of her needle and after binds up the little wound with a hollow bit of shell. In this manner she opens four or five veins.

MRS. MURRAY What happens? What is the result of this gruesome practice?

LADY MARY   They are well for eight days. Then the fever seizes them and they keep to their beds two days – seldom three. They have rarely more than twenty or thirty pustules on their face, which leave no mark, and then they are as well as before their inoculation.

MRS. MURRAY Does no one die from this contrived smallpox?

LADY MARY   There is no example of any one having died. You may believe I am very well satisfied in the safety of the experiment since I intend to try it on my own dear little son.

MRS. MURRAY But my dear, I protest. Do but consider ...

*   *   *

At the time, Lady Mary's news of the technique of putting pus into a wound, a technique known as *inoculation,* caused less comment than the fact that she had brought home a mummy, or that she had dined with the Sultana and been bored or had visited the beautiful Fatima, wife of the powerful Deputy to the Vizier. The gossip about Lady Mary was second only to gossip about the Prince of Wales. If gossip was an ocean, her return to London created a tidal wave. "Not to have been to her informal receptions, where her more intimate friends of both sexes could finger her Turkish costumes, goggle at her foreign servants, price her new lace, new knick-knacks, and new jewels and watch her – in the hands of her maid and her good-looking Italian valet-de-chambre and hairdresser – being embellished for the day, was to be utterly unfashionable."[7]

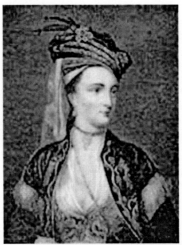

Lady Mary Wortley Montagu in Turkish dress.

Princess Caroline, daughter-in-law of George I and later queen of England, was impressed by Lady Mary's assertions, and determined to test inoculation. In the summer of 1721 six condemned prisoners in Newgate were allowed to volunteer for the operation, with freedom as their reward. Five of the six developed a mild attack of smallpox and the sixth, who had previously had smallpox, showed no change. Encouraged, the Princess had a group of orphans inoculated. While the criminals were pardoned as a reward for their participation, the orphans received the satisfaction of making a contribution to science and were rewarded, in some instances, with blindness, lameness and death.[8] After grave consideration and more than a few protestations of horror, the Royal children and Lady Mary's daughter were inoculated.

Just as royalty and the famous set the fashion today so they did in the 1700s and the idea of inoculation spread among the upper classes. Then two people died: a young servant in a Lord's household and the small son of the Earl of Sutherland.[9] The church deplored the intervention in God's will, physicians deplored the influence of "ignorant women" and the public deplored the spread of the disease. Lady Mary took to her pen, not to write poetry as usual, but to write an essay, *"A Plain Account of the Inoculating of the Small Pox by a Turkey Merchant."*

---

[7] Barry, Iris. *Portrait of Lady Mary Wortley Montagu.* Ernest Menn Ltd. 1928

[8] Hale, AR. *The Medical Voodoo.* Gotham House Inc. 1935

[9] Halsband, Robert. *The Life of Lady Mary Wortley Montagu.* Clarendon Press, 1956

I suppose it's not a bad idea really, to give yourself a disease at a convenient time. However the upper classes who embraced the practice had the luxury of clean beds, food and servants to care for them, while those of the lower classes who contracted the disease from them would not be so fortunate. Inoculation was not, of course, a cure or preventative for smallpox as it induced an active case of the disease. The trouble was that inoculated people were fully contagious during their brief illness so that they could, and did, start epidemics.

Dr. Lettsom, writing in 1806, tells us that whereas smallpox deaths for 42 years before inoculation were 72 per thousand, there were 89 per thousand in the 42 years after its introduction.[10] Furthermore, conscientious physicians could see a connection between inoculation and the increased incidence of worse diseases than smallpox, such as syphilis, tuberculosis and erysipelas.

Councillor Asbury, Chairman of Sheffield's Health Committee, wrote in 1927: "It has been calculated that from 1721 to 1758 smallpox inoculation was responsible for the deaths of no less than 22,700 persons from smallpox in London alone. It is not therefore surprising that when Jenner proposed that smallpox inoculation should be given up and cowpox inoculation substituted for it – thus covering the retreat of the (medical) profession from an untenable position, his ideas were accepted by all whose interests were not conspicuously bound up with the older form of treatment."[11]

Eventually in 1840 an Act of Parliament was passed forbidding the practice of inoculation, largely because, as Asbury mentions, Edward Jenner had offered an alternative.

---

[10] Hadwen, W. *The Case Against Vaccination.*, Verbatim report of an address given at Goddards Assembly Rooms, Gloucester, January 25, 1896
[11] Hale, AR. *The Medical Voodoo.* Gotham House Inc. 1935

Chapter 3

Edward Jenner

Precursors of today's pharmacists were apothecaries, who themselves started as wholesale merchants and spice importers. They grew in numbers in the 17th century to the point where the Royal College of Physicians became concerned about their power. This College, founded as a learned society by a royal charter of Henry VIII in 1518, would obtain the right to inspect the wares of apothecaries by an Act of 1553. In 1617 the College succeeded in separating the apothecaries from the Grocers' Company and the Worshipful Society of Apothecaries was formed.

In the following year, 1618, the College published an official pharmacopoeia which specified the drugs apothecaries were allowed to dispense. As well as controlling drugs, the College sought to fine or imprison unlicensed practitioners or upstart apothecaries for practising any kind of medicine.[12] These practitioners included herbalists, midwives and 'wise women' who tended the sick in their communities. An Act of Parliament in 1542, (disparagingly known as the 'Quacks' charter), allowed the latter people to practice but only on condition that their services were free of charge.

Since the 17th century physicians through governments have exerted control over other health care providers and continue to do so today. Only recently have midwives been allowed to practice in Canada; other alternative practitioners there are successfully controlled by not allowing them to bill through government medical insurance schemes.

Edward Jenner was born in 1749 and died in 1823.[13] At 14 years old he was apprenticed to an apothecary and surgeon. In Jenner's time surgeons were nothing like modern surgeons. The United Company of Barber-Surgeons had been formed in 1540 and its members were legally restricted to setting bones, healing outward wounds with topical preparations, carrying out bleeding and undertaking the limited operations in this pre-anaesthetic era, such as amputations and removal of bladder stones.[14] It is in recognition of the past association with barbers that British Fellows of the Royal College of Surgeons relinquish the title of 'Doctor' for that of 'Mister'.

---

[12] Tobyn, Graeme, *Culpeppers' Medicine*. Element Books Ltd. 1997
[13] www.jennermuseum.com
[14] Ibid

Edward Jenner, the son of a prosperous family in the Church who owned a small landed estate, grew up in the Gloucestershire countryside where he enjoyed the study of natural history. In 1788 he was elected as a Fellow of the Royal Society, not because of his experiments with cowpox, as some writers would have us believe, but because of a paper he wrote, "*The Natural History of the Cuckoo.*"

Jenner set up practice as a surgeon in Berkeley but despite the description of him as a country physician he did not earn the title of "doctor". A contemporary of Jenner's, Walter Hadwen, JP, MD, LRCP, MRCS, LSA., said during an address in 1896, of which a verbatim report exists, "Now this man Jenner had never passed a medical examination in his life. He belonged to the good old times when George III was King, when medical examinations were not compulsory. Jenner looked upon the whole thing as a superfluity ... It was not until twenty years after he was in practice that he thought it advisable to get a few letters after his name. Consequently he communicated with a Scotch university and obtained the degree of Doctor of Medicine for the sum of £15 and nothing more.

"A few years after this, rather dissatisfied with the only medical qualification he had obtained, Jenner communicated with the University of Oxford and asked them to grant him their honorary degree of MD and after a good many fruitless attempts he got it. Then he sent to the Royal College of Physicians in London to get their diploma, and even presented his Oxford degree as an argument in his favour. But they considered he had had quite enough on the cheap already, and told him distinctly that until he passed the usual examinations they were not going to give him any more. This was a sufficient check in Jenner's case, and he settled down quietly without any diploma of physician." [15]

Living in rural Gloucestershire, Jenner would have known the local superstition that those who contracted cowpox did not get smallpox. How the superstition arose is dealt with at length by Dr. Charles Creighton in *Jenner and Vaccination: a Strange Chapter of Medical History,* published in 1889. [16] In this book Creighton says, "The single bond connecting cowpox with smallpox was the occurrence of the word "pox" in each name; it was a case of the river in Macedon and the river in Monmouth. The jingle of the names had the effect that it often has upon credulous people, whose acquaintance with any matter is more verbal than real." Creighton also goes on to observe: "To a pathologist or epidemiologist, it is as truly nonsense to speak of cowpox becoming smallpox as it is legitimate nonsense to prove that a horse-chestnut is a chestnut horse. It was reserved for Edward Jenner to take up that surprising legend, and make it scientifically passable, despite the impatience and ridicule which his prosaic medical neighbours in the cowpox districts had met it with."

Cowpox is a disease that occurs on the teats of cows only when they are in milk. The causative virus is said to be *orthopox vaccinia*; it results in an ugly

---

[15] Hadwen, Walter. *The Case Against Vaccination*, Verbatim report of an address given at Goddards Assembly Rooms, Gloucester, January 25, 1896
[16] Creighton, C. *Jenner and Vaccination: a Strange Chapter of Medical History.* Swan Sonnerschein & Co. 1889. Found on www.whale/to

chancre; it is not infectious; it is, of course, found only in female animals. People who milked infected animals developed pustules on their hands, which in turn, led to swollen glands and general malaise.

Smallpox, on the other hand, is not limited to the female sex nor to one portion of the body. The causative virus is said to be *orthopox variola*; it is found only in humans; it is highly infectious.[17]

There is no correspondence between cowpox and smallpox as legitimate scientists of Jenner's day, such as Crookshank, Hadwen and Wallace, were well aware. Nevertheless, based on the superstition of dairymaids, Jenner proceeded to experiment on an eight-year old boy, James Phipps, by inserting cowpox pus from a dairymaid, Sarah Nelmes. into his body. The scene is imagined, the events real.

*   *   *

Sarah hides her hands under her apron so that she won't scratch the itching sores that cover them. She is due to leave the farm in a few minutes to meet with Edward Jenner, a local apothecary and surgeon and she doesn't want to go. "Mother, you should never of told him I'd go. Not without asking me."

"He's paying three pence."

Sarah shrugs and raises her eyes.

Her father says sternly, "You have no milking duties today, Sarah. Now leave or you'll be late." He is not a man to defy.

Sarah adjusts her mob cap over her long dark curls, ties a clean apron over her blue dress, and sets off to walk the mile to Berkeley. It is a gloomy May day; May 14 1796, to be exact. Several days of ceaseless rain have made the track muddy and, after sliding a few times, Sarah regrets wearing her best frock.

The apothecary's house is a square brick establishment set in the middle of the village. A housekeeper answers Sarah's knock and ushers her into Jenner's drawing room. "Sarah Nelmes, sir."

Sarah curtsies to the heavy-set man who rises to greet her. Although he smiles she does not take to the loose mouth, the plump cheeks or the soft, fair hair that hangs limply over his collar. Nor to the way he turns her hands back and forth as he examines her pustules.

"Good, good," he says. "Now, where's the boy?"

Sarah hears a scuffle in the hall before the housekeeper drags in a small boy dressed in knickerbockers and a loose shirt. "Ah, James," Jenner says. "This is Sarah who has the cowpox. That is what I propose to give you so you won't get the smallpox, for people who have had the cowpox do not get the smallpox. Is that not correct, Sarah?"

"So they say, sir. But I do know a lad who had both."

"That cannot happen," Jenner says brusquely. "Now James, I am going to make scratches on your arm and then put in some matter from Sarah's sores."

---

[17] O'Shea, T. *The Sanctity of Human Blood: Vaccination I$ not Immunization.* Two Trees, San Jose, California, 2004

James attempts to bolt but the housekeeper holds him firmly and pushes his unwilling body over to where Jenner is sitting, his instruments beside him. "Roll up your sleeves, boy," Jenner commands.

With unnecessary force the housekeeper drags up James's sleeve and holds out his left arm. The lancet incises two or three cuts on his lower arm, deep enough to draw blood. James begins to cry.

"Now Sarah, give me your hand."

She reluctantly holds out her hand. The lancet flicks closer and closer and she shudders with the anticipation of pain. A sharp stab that stings like a wasp and the largest pustule oozes out its contents: cream-coloured pus that threatens to drip on to the Turkish carpet. Sarah turns her eyes away and scans the elegant room with its painting of a nymph, its velvet curtains and the leering jovial face of a Toby jug.

Jenner inserts a metal spatula into the pus and spreads it over the cuts in James's arm. Sarah watches in disbelief. It is bad enough that she got the cowpox from milking infected cows but to deliberately give it to a child? She looks for other signs of madness in Edward Jenner but he has his back to her as he bandages James's arm. The housekeeper hands Sarah a cloth to place on her oozing hand.

"Now the other arm," Jenner says. Sarah closes her eyes as he tears the flesh of the child's other arm and then jabs at two more of her sores. This time he holds her hand close to James's arm as he scrapes the pus on to the boy. His hand is hot and rough.

Finally the bandaged boy and the shaken dairy maid are free to go. "You will come out in the pox in a few days," Jenner says to James. "You may feel ill. But see how Sarah thrives. One day, you will thank me for saving you from the ravages of smallpox."

*   *   *

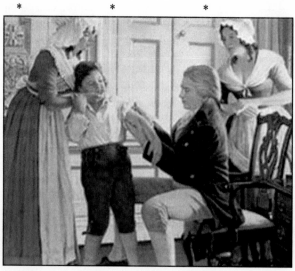

Two months later, on July 1st, 1796, Jenner made more incisions into the arms of James Phipps, age 8, but this time he smeared the cuts with smallpox pus. The boy did not contract smallpox. As no figures were kept in this unscientific era it is impossible to say whether insertion of smallpox pus under the skin inevitably produced a case of smallpox. Many people, including children, were immune to smallpox anyway having encountered it without developing a case of the disease. When I started nurse training we were all tested for tuberculosis. Most of us were immune even though we had never had the disease.

On the basis of this experiment with a *single subject*, the practice of vaccination was born.

James Phipps was re-vaccinated 20 times. Jenner's biographer, Baron, relates that while walking with a friend they passed Phipps and Jenner remarked, "Oh, there is poor Phipps! I wish you could see him. He has been very unwell lately and I am afraid he has got tubercles in his lungs. He was recently inoculated for smallpox, I believe for the twentieth time, and all without effect."[18]

Some writers claim that James Phipps died from tuberculosis at the age of twenty-one but one source states that he recovered and lived until 1853.[19] Jenner's son, who was also vaccinated more than once, died at twenty-one from tuberculosis. Tuberculosis is a condition that some researchers have linked to the smallpox vaccine.[20] In fact, Dr. A. Wilder, Professor of Pathology and former editor of *The New York Medical Times*, went so far as to say, "Consumption (TB) follows in the wake of vaccination as surely as effect follows cause."[21]

Jenner continued with his experiments and in 1798 wrote about them, describing each case in detail. He continued to promote the idea that cowpox prevented smallpox. "Morbid matter of various kinds, when absorbed into the system, may produce effects in some degree similar; but what renders the cowpox virus so extremely singular is that the person who has been thus affected is forever secure from the infection of the smallpox; neither exposure to the various effluvia, nor the insertion of the matter into the skin, producing the distemper."[22]

Jenner is not using the word "virus" to mean a smaller-than-a light-wave inert particle of protein and genetic code as we normally understand it now in biology but to mean a "poison or venom;" the Latin for "poison" being "virus".

Not everyone agreed with him. He wrote in a later paper, "I have lately been favoured with a letter from a gentleman of great respectability (Dr. Ingenhousz), informing me that, on making an inquiry into the subject in the county of Wilts, he discovered that a farmer near Calne had been infected with the smallpox after

---

[18] Hale, AR. *The Medical Voodoo*. Gotham House Inc. 1935
[19] Cohn, DV. James Phipps. www.founderofscience.net/Phipps.htm
[20] Miller, N.Z. *Vaccines: Are They Really Safe and Effective?* New Atlantean Press, New Mexico, 1992
[21] Rattigan, P. Assault on the Species, *Truth Campaign Magazine*, 15
[22] Jenner, E. *An Inquiry into the Causes and Effects of the Variolae Vaccine*. 1798. www.whale.to/a/jenner4.htm

having had the cowpox and that the disease in each instance was so strongly characterized as to render the facts incontrovertible." [23]

Other physicians told him the same thing but unwilling to believe that his theory was false, he called these cases of smallpox, "spurious cowpox." Undaunted, he looked for another source of vaccine and found it in the oozing pus of infected horses' heels, a condition known as "grease". His reasoning about why grease was the precursor of cowpox makes interesting reading

"From the similarity of symptoms, both constitutional and local, between the cow-pox and the disease received from morbid matter generated by a horse, the common people in this neighbourhood, when infected with this disease, through a strange perversion of terms, frequently call it the cow-pox. Let us suppose, then, such a malady to appear among some of the servants at a farm, and at the same time that the cow-pox were to break out among the cattle; and let us suppose, too, that some of the servants were infected in this way, and that others received the infection from the cows. It would be recorded at the farm, and among the servants themselves wherever they might afterwards be dispersed, that they had all had the cow-pox. But it is clear that an individual thus infected from the horse would neither be for a certainty secure himself, nor would he impart smallpox. Yet were this to happen before the nature of the cowpox be more maturely considered by the public my evidence on the subject might be depreciated unjustly."

I think he is saying that there is another form of cowpox and that it is horse-grease cowpox and he is attempting to discriminate between them so that he can use the pus from the horse's heels for his vaccine. But the public was appalled and given a choice, preferred the diseased secretions from cows' teats over the oozing pus from horses' heels.

Variolation, introduced by Lady Mary, was still going strong and Jenner used the opportunity to deliver people from "the inconveniences, uncertainties, disasters, and horrors of variolation."[24] He petitioned the House of Commons in 1802, and again in 1807, for large sums of money to promote smallpox vaccinations, promising that his product had the "singularly beneficial effect of rendering through life the person so inoculated perfectly secure from the infection of smallpox."[25]

Parliament granted his request by a vote of 59 to 56 and gave him the equivalent of half a million of today's dollars. I often reflect on the narrowness of this majority vote and how different public health would be had the figures been reversed.

Vaccination campaigns began. It didn't take long before cases of smallpox among the vaccinated were reported. The first response was denial but when the vaccinated were obviously afflicted, Jenner and his supporters said that the disease was milder in form. But when the vaccinated caught the disease and died, they had

---

[23] Jenner, E. *Further Observations on the Variolae Vaccina, of Cow-pox.* www.whale.to/a/jenner4.htm

[24] Ibid.

[25] Ibid.

to come up with another explanation. Re-naming the disease did the trick – they didn't die of smallpox, they died of the re-named disease: spurious cowpox.

Despite *increasing evidence* that vaccination with cowpox pus did not prevent smallpox, the practice continued. Physicians, for the first time, attended the healthy; 100% of their catchment areas could now be treated instead of the 10% who had contracted smallpox. As Dr. Hadwen so aptly remarked in 1896, "What Jenner discovered, though hardly original in its general principle, was that it pays far better to scare 100% of the fools in the world – the vast majority – into buying vaccine than it does to treat the small minority who really get smallpox and who cannot afford to pay anything. It was indeed a very great discovery – worth thousands of millions. That is why this kind of blackmail is still kept going." [26]

Royalty was again particularly enthusiastic about vaccination. In 1811, the Empress of Russia presented Jenner with a diamond ring and had the first child vaccinated in her empire named "Vaccinoff."[27]

When Jenner died in 1823, three kinds of smallpox vaccines were in use: 1) cowpox –promoted as "pure lymph from the calf," 2) horsegrease – promoted as "the true and genuine life-preserving fluid," and 3) horse-grease cowpox.[28]

Following Jenner's death the vaccine establishment used one excuse after another to explain the failure of vaccination: the number of punctures was incorrect, or that re-vaccination was necessary or that the lymph was impure. The deaths of vaccinated patients in hospital were recorded as "pustular eczema."

Neil Miller, in *Immunization: Theory vs. Reality,*[29] devised a flow chart to show how a campaign to eradicate smallpox took place:

- Begin with – unsanitary conditions and poor nutritional awareness.
- This results in – regional and self-limiting outbreaks of smallpox.
- Conduct human experiments with – variolation.
- When this fails – conduct human experiments with cowpox, horse-grease cowpox.
- When this fails – deny it.
- When this fails – recommend revaccination.
- When this fails – manipulate statistics by re-naming the disease.
- When everyone begins catching on, and vaccination rates drop, and cases of smallpox dwindle – take full credit for eradicating the disease.

---

[26] Hadwen, W. *The Case Against Vaccination.*, Verbatim report of an address given at Goddards Assembly Rooms, Gloucester, January 25, 1896
[27] Hale, AR. *The Medical Voodoo.* Gotham House Inc. 1935
[28] Miller, NZ. *Immunization: Theory vs. Reality.* New Atlantean Press, Santa Fe, New Mexico, 1996
[29] Ibid.

Chapter 4

Vaccine Manufacturing

About fifteen miles from Berkeley, where Jenner practised as an apothecary and surgeon, lies Randwick, a tiny village set among farms and woods. In 1940 Randwick boasted a church, a shop, a school and a few stone cottages. My mother, brother and I were sent to live in Randwick Vicarage when German bombs began to pulverize Coventry's engineering works.

The vicar was some sort of uncle, the threads of kinship lost somewhere in death and re-marriage. The matriarch of the vicarage, Auntie as I called her, was small, rotund, energetic, – and intolerant of childishness in me, my brother, her four children, and the Jewish boy they rescued from Czechoslovakia. My favourite memory of her is in a tin hat with a garden rake over one shoulder lined up with neighbours, similarly armed, and prepared to fight on the beaches, on the landing grounds and in the hills. They would never surrender. Neither would we children although, at six years old, I wasn't quite sure what the word meant.

Fields became our playgrounds; stone walls, oak trees and gates our climbing equipment. Whenever I had the chance I would skip down the narrow lane – I was a very skippy child – to visit my friends at the Godsell's farm. I liked to gather bouquets of wild flowers from the lush hedgerows or to make dolls out of red poppies or to weave daisy chains from the white carpet that surrounded the farm house. It was at this farm that I learned to play croquet and tennis, ride a pony and chase rats out of the barn into the jaws of waiting dogs. I also learned about birth. As though on cue for a children's show, a cow produced a calf and we watched in awe as she licked her baby and nudged him to his feet. I fell in love with Adolf, as we called him, and delighted in stroking his rough forehead and feeling the slobbery softness of his mouth.

Such familiarity with the Gloucestershire countryside makes it easy to see the setting in which Jenner practiced as, at that time, there had been little change in the rural nature of the area. It is easy to imagine a dairymaid in a white mob-cap, long dress and apron, leading a small calf by a rope down a grassy path towards Berkeley.

*   *   *

"Do you bring the heifer then?" Tom calls to Daisy from his shed.

"Aye, Mr.Tom. As you said, 18 weeks old. But what does he want with it? A whole shilling to borrow a calf?"

"Dunno, Daisy." Tom rubs his chin. "We'll find out soon enough. He said he wants to make a vaccine. Here he comes."

Daisy watches as a burly man in breeches and a plum-coloured jacket approaches on horseback and dismounts heavily.

"Mr. Jenner, this be Daisy, the dairymaid from down the way." Daisy curtsies.

Jenner nods at her. "You brought a calf then? A heifer? Good. I shall only need it for ten days. Today I perform the first operation." He looks around him. "You have the board? Good. Now you must tie the animal to it."

Tom and Daisy struggle with the small heifer which frantically resists their efforts to lie it down on the board. Not until Jenner holds its head are they able to secure the flailing legs with ropes and attach them to the hooks Tom had nailed into the board. Except for its rolling eyes, the calf is still.

"You have the razor, soap and water, Tom?"

"Aye, sir."

"Right. Now I want you to wash and shave its belly from here to here." Jenner indicates the area between the forelegs and the tail.

Daisy strokes the calf's forehead as Tom lathers the belly and then opens the razor to shave it. Jenner watches for a moment and then wanders outside and adjusts the harness of his horse before removing two wrapped packages from the saddle bag.

"All done, sir," Tom calls.

Jenner lays his packages on the ground beside the helpless calf. From one he extracts a lancet and proceeds to make small nicks in the shaved skin of the belly. Daisy gasps and turns her head away. After Jenner has made about 50 incisions, he opens the second package and prises the lid off a porcelain jar.

"What's that?" Daisy wrinkles her nose and lifts her hand to her nostrils.

"Pus. Matter from the very best cowpox," Jenner says. He dips a narrow, metal spatula into the yellow pus and touches each incision with it. Back and forth goes the spatula from dish to incision until all cuts have received a drop of pus.

Daisy feels sick. She continues to stroke the calf's head and keeps her eyes away from the belly.

At last Jenner finishes. Tom and Daisy release the calf which struggles to its feet.

"Now, Daisy, I want you to pen this animal so that it cannot lick its underside. Do you understand?"

"Aye, sir."

"Do you have a suitable pen? One that will hold its head?"

"I do, sir."

"Excellent. Now, when the pustules are ripe for squeezing, you are to bring the beast back here. That will be, let me see, a week Thursday. Can you do that?"

"Aye, sir." Daisy picks up the rope that holds the calf by its neck.

"Have you had the cowpox, my girl?" Jenner asks her.

"Aye, sir. More'n once."

"And have you had the smallpox?"

"I have not."

"There, you see." Jenner turns triumphantly to Tom. "Persons who have had the cowpox cannot get the smallpox."

"So they say, sir. But I do know one fellow who had both. Left he very scarred."

"He probably had chicken pox. Or pustular eczema. It's easy to confuse them."

"Aye, so you say, sir." Tom raises his eyebrows at Daisy.

Daisy walks the calf home and secures it in the special pen her father had made. When she looks at the poor inflamed belly she wonders if the damage was worth the shilling. She had helped with this calf's birth. At first, the baby animal lay lifeless in the straw until she had cleaned out her mouth and rubbed her body vigorously. Then the calf had struggled to her feet to be licked by her mother before suckling. Daisy sighs. Twelve pence was a lot of money, money the family needed.

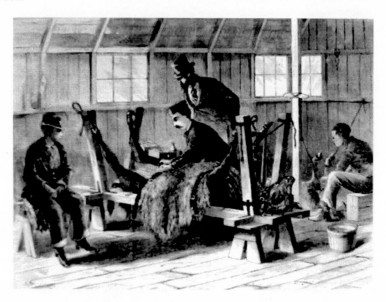

Ten days later Daisy leads the calf back to Tom's shed, slowly this time as the little animal can barely walk. Nor does it have the strength to resist as they tie it down on the board. They wait for Jenner. Daisy cannot bear to look at the inflamed belly covered with pustules; fifty of them; one yellow, festering sore on each of the incisions Jenner had made. She had once had a boil on the back of her neck and she remembers how painful it was.

Jenner rolls up his sleeves before he examines the calf. He produces the tools he needs: a clamp, a lancet and a crucible. Starting at one end of a row of pustules he systematically works on each by bursting it with the clamp and scraping the pus, blood and scab into the crucible.

Daisy closes her eyes and strokes the calf. She tries to think of the penny her mother has promised her and the colour of the satin ribbon she will buy with it.

Should it be pink to match the roses in her summer bonnet or blue to go with her flowered dress? Pink or blue, she repeats to herself, pink or blue?

"*What's that muck furr?*" *Tom asks Jenner.*

"*I shall mix it with an equal quantity of glycerine,*" *Jenner says without looking up,* "*strain it and the result will save hundreds of lives.*"

"*Oh, aye.*"

"*Yes. I shall place a drop of this mixture into an incision I shall make in a patient's arm.*"

"*Oh, aye. And what will that do?*"

"*It will prevent smallpox, my man. No smallpox. Think of it.*"

*   *   *

But that was in 1796 and we have advanced a great deal since then. NOVA, a science program on the USA's Public Broadcasting Station, explains on its website how to make a smallpox vaccine. "To create a vaccine that will protect you against a pathogen, you usually begin with that pathogen and alter it in some way. Not so with smallpox. To create this vaccine, you begin with another virus that is similar to the smallpox virus, yet different enough not to bring on the smallpox disease once it enters your body. This similar virus is cowpox!"

The idea that the cowpox virus will protect you against smallpox is still alive and well today despite our knowledge of microbiology, DNA and immunology. And this is not just on a science program for children. The Centers for Diseases Control (CDC) has a Smallpox Fact Sheet on its website. Under the heading, 'Facts about vaccinia' two of the seven points are:

1. The vaccinia virus, the virus in the smallpox vaccine, is another "pox" type virus,
2. The vaccinia is related to smallpox, but milder.[30]

The big question I have is this: why is the smallpox vaccine the only one without the correct causative agent? Cowpox is said to be caused by a virus called *orthopox vaccinia*, smallpox by a virus called *orthopox variola*. Why isn't the smallpox vaccine made with *orthopox variola*? If the basic axioms of immunology are true, how can one disease vector immunize against a completely separate disease?

The NOVA article continues with a picture of a cow with a spotted udder and the caption: "The cow has been intentionally infected with cowpox virus. The fluid you collect from virus-caused pustules on the cow's udder contains many copies of the virus."

But what else does it contain? Pus from the cowpox pustule could conceivably contain the virus not only of cowpox but also of tuberculosis, syphilis, gonorrhoea and anthrax.

So far the method described by NOVA is not much different from Jenner's, but wait: today you use a purifier to isolate the viruses. This purification process is

---

[30] www.cdc.gov/smallpox

illustrated by a picture of a square, metal box with a funnel in the top and a tap protruding from one side. A squiggle indicates that you pour the pus into the funnel and it emerges out of the tap into a beaker, all ready to be injected. A syringe is poised above the beaker. The caption reads: "The smallpox vaccine is a live vaccine; the cowpox viruses it contains will invade cells in your body, multiply, and spread to other cells in your body, just as the smallpox viruses would. And as with smallpox, the body's immune system will mount an attack against the cowpox and subsequently always "remember" what it looks like. Then, if cowpox or the similar smallpox ever enters the body, the immune system will quickly get rid of the invaders."

This article is written for students. My children grew up in West Vancouver, British Columbia, an area not noted for pastures. I am surely glad that they did not have the desire to make a smallpox vaccine, as I would have been hard pressed to find a cow with or without an infected udder.

Vaccines, other than smallpox, are made with three categories of ingredients: cultured bacteria or viruses, the medium or "substrate" in which the bacteria or virus is produced, and the stabilizer or neutralizer.

The first ingredient is cultured bacteria or viruses which are thought to be the cause of the infectious disease the vaccine is supposed to prevent. Sometimes the bacteria or viruses are attenuated which means weakened.

However, all viruses, even those that are called "killed" or "attenuated", are made by cells and contain inert RNA or DNA which is "shed" when the virus is broken up or absorbed by other cells.

One theory is that viral DNA or RNA can lie dormant in tissues throughout the body and be activated at a later stage, sometimes years later, triggering auto-immune responses. Auto-immune diseases result when the body attacks itself, as if it cannot distinguish between foreign invaders and its own tissues.[31] But, I must confess I do not yet know what happens to the viruses or bacteria in vaccines after they have entered the body. It seems from reviewing the scientific literature that many scientists are still unsure about what precisely happens to them.

The second category of ingredient in vaccine preparation is the medium. Cells of all kinds, including bacterial, are grown in warm incubators. If viruses are wanted, the cells are stressed or poisoned to persuade them to make the required viruses. The cells used, the 'media' or 'substrate', as listed in the *Physicians Desk Reference,* can be the lung cells of an aborted foetus, kidneys or testicles of monkeys, infected animal cells (monkey, pig, calf, canary, chicken, guinea pig), and human blood or infected human connective tissue. These cells may also be deliberately "immortalized" or made cancerous. As these cells get sick and die, the vaccine incubators are inevitably contaminated with many foreign proteins, enzymes and genetic codes from the decomposing cellular waste. I was shocked to discover that the smaller elements of this cannot be filtered from the vaccines - and thus are injected directly into the bloodstream of children.

---

[31] Null, G. *Vaccines: a Second Opinion.* www.garynull.com

Vaccine suspensions are derived from the manufacturer's 'incubation tanks' in which the viruses are produced from mashed bird embryo, minced monkey kidneys or cloned human cells. These suspensions are filtered before use but only to remove particles larger than viruses. The point of the vaccine is that it contains viruses, so these must not be filtered out. Therefore, anything smaller than a virus remains.

These remains include what the vaccine manufacturers call 'degradation products' – parts of decayed viruses or cells, unknown bits and pieces, foreign protein particles, viral oncogenes (might cause cancer), added chemicals and DNA fragments.[32]

Under normal circumstances, ingested substances have to pass through the mucus membranes of the mouth and other orifices, the intestinal walls or the liver, before they are permitted into such important organs as the heart or the brain. The sudden appearance of a poison in the bloodstream via injection is met by a counterattack from the immune system, one designed to prevent sudden death or an allergic response. The counterattack does not always succeed; anaphylactic shock sometimes follows vaccination.

Undigested proteins in the blood are one of the causes of allergies and furthermore, undigested proteins can attack the myelin sheath that protects the nerves and results in neurological damage.

How to remove contaminating DNA has caused some concern to the Authorities which is comforting. In 1986, the US government recommended a weight limit of 100 picograms of contaminating DNA per vaccine dose. However, this has proved so impossible a standard to achieve that they now allow one hundred times that amount, i.e. 10 nanograms per vaccine dose.[33]

Monkey kidneys are the preferred medium for growing polio viruses. From the 1950's tens of thousands of Rhesus and African Green monkeys were killed for this purpose, with chimpanzees used widely for "safety testing" experiments.

Two eminent virologists, Dr. B. H. Sweet and Dr. M. R. Hilleman, found that both the Salk and Sabin vaccines were contaminated with a monkey virus – simian virus 40, or SV40.[34] Furthermore, two research papers written by Eddy et al. and Girardi et al. reported that SV40 virus causes tumours in hamsters.[35] In the 1990s this same virus was discovered in human bone cancers, in brain tumours among children and in human mesotheliomas. In fact, anyone who got polio vaccine, including me, has been probably exposed to SV40.

According to Dr. John Martin of the Center for Complex Infectious Diseases, SV40 infection has been observed in 23% of blood samples taken from normal

---

[32] Roberts, J. *Fear of the Invisible*. Impact Investigative Media Productions, 2008
[33] Roberts, J. *Fear of the Invisible*. Impact Investigative Media Productions, 2008
[34] Snicer, A. Near disaster with the Salk vaccine. *Science Digest*, December, 1963
[35] Scheibner, V. *Vaccination: 100 Years of Orthodox Research Shows that Vaccination Represents a Medical Assault on the Immune System*. New Atlantean Press, 1993 p.155

individuals.[36] Furthermore, the virus can be detected in sperm fluid and is likely to be passed congenitally to future generations.

To give them credit, in 1973 the *Medical Journal of Australia* did warn people about the contamination: "To date more than 40 separate simian viruses have been isolated from this tissue, (monkey kidney). They include virus B, known to cause encephalitis in man, and SV40, which can produce cancer in hamsters, as well as changes in human cell tissue cultures. There has been no sign so far that vaccines grown on primary monkey kidney tissue produce alarming symptoms; but symptoms may not appear for 20 years or more."[37]

It was thought that all SV40 was removed from the vaccine by 1964, but it has since been revealed that it was never successfully totally removed and that every single dose of polio vaccine up to recent years has remained contaminated with from 100 to 10,000 monkey viruses.[38]

The British Medical Journal in 1998 reported that SV40 has re-emerged as a potentially oncogenic (cancer producing) virus, confirming that SV40 has been identified in human tumours such as osteosarcomas (bone tumours) and malignant deadly mesotheliomas. However, although they say "it remains possible that a late adverse effect of the polio vaccination programme is emerging," they modify the statement by saying, "*any risk of cancer is likely to be more than outweighed by the benefit of vaccination to the postwar generation.*"

Benefit? Who is to decide the relative risk? Would people undergoing cancer treatment today agree that the previous polio vaccination program was worth this 'late adverse effect'?

The vaccines we inject into our children are not composed of selected viruses in a sterile fluid to which preservatives have been added but are liquids filled with unknown particles, most of which come from cells of non-humans: from chickens, monkeys, and even from cancer cells, and thus include the *DNA of other species*.

The third category of ingredient in vaccine preparation is the stabilizer, neutralizer, carrying agent or preservative.

There are some smells that, if I experienced them today, transport me back to my nurse training days in the fifties. I don't mean human smells, and god knows there were plenty of those, I mean the sort of distinctive pungency that settles in the throat and that you can identify at once. Carbolic acid, for example.

We used carbolic, a pink fluid contained in bottles marked *Poison*, to disinfect anything from sputum mugs to bedpans to rubber draw sheets. An oblong piece of tough, red rubber was held on the bed, under the draw sheet, by two attached lengths of sheeting. They were for incontinent patients, those with oozing dressings and anyone emitting any type of body fluid. Washing 'macs', as we called them, was an evening chore for the most junior nurse. We had to wash the rubber with carbolic and the sheet part with soap and then hang it to dry on a

---

[36] http://ccid.org
[37] Sinclair, I. *Vaccination: The "Hidden" Facts*. Australia, 1992
[38] Roberts. J. Ibid. page 33.

pulley over the bath tub. As a junior nurse my hands were usually red, rough and sore from prolonged contact with carbolic acid.

Another distinctive smell was that of formaldehyde. Nurses did not dissect the cadavers that were preserved in this fluid but we were asked to observe and examine things like gall stones, diseased kidneys or deformed babies that were housed in jars of formaldehyde in the pathology department. I always thought that the instructors were unnecessarily gleeful as they demonstrated these specimens; they seemed to relish our disgust at both the sight and the smell.

Those were the days when we took a patient's temperature with a glass rod that contained mercury. Once the column of mercury had risen to display the temperature, it was very difficult to shake down. Nurses developed a decisive wrist flick, one that distinguished the expert from the novice. New nurses tried all sorts of wild arm motions that often ended with broken glass and little globs of mercury. We had no idea that this metal is toxic. I remember playing with the erratic silver balls on a patient's bed table in much the same way as one plays with spilt salt in a restaurant. I can't remember how we disposed of it once we had captured it – probably in the general garbage.

The *Physicians Desk Reference* informs us of the ingredients used as preservatives in the production of vaccines. These include:

Formaldehyde – a known cancer-causing agent that is commonly used to embalm corpses. It is in the current polio vaccine.

Phenol (carbolic acid) – a deadly poison.

Thimerosal (a mercury derivative) – a toxic, heavy metal that is not easily eliminated by the body, found in certain flu vaccines, among others.

Acetone – a solvent used in nail polish remover that is volatile and can easily cross the placental barrier.

Aluminium phosphate – used in deodorants and has been connected with Alzheimer's disease.

Glycerine – tri-atomic alcohol derived from decomposed fats which can damage kidney, liver, lungs and local tissue.

From the start, vaccine manufacturers have been obsessed with animal tissue, and infected animal tissue at that. Have they never thought about DNA transfer? Is the practice of injecting our children with fluids and viruses from monkey kidneys, passed through chick embryos and cultured in an embalming fluid, really good for their health? Is there any evidence that this practice prevents disease? What becomes of these foreign substances once they are inside the body?

Vaccines are tested for potency by injecting five samples into 350-400 mice. If the vaccine creates antibodies in the majority of these mice, it is said that it will do the same in humans, even if the antibodies are different, and thus it is released for use.[39]

---

[39] Coulter, HL & Fisher, BL. *A Shot in the Dark.* Avery Publishing Group Inc. 1991

Tests for toxicity, meaning how likely is the vaccine to cause severe reactions in children, are also performed on young mice. The vaccine is injected into the abdominal cavities of the mice to see if they will continue to gain weight over time. If they do not die and if they gain a specific amount of weight, the vaccine manufacturers and the FDA, (US Food and Drug Administration) consider the vaccine safe. The mouse-weight test is the *only* safety test that has ever been done on the DPT vaccine in the past fifty years.[40]

The usual controlled trials, where one group receives the drug and the other a placebo, considered to be the gold standard for drug safety trials, are not conducted with vaccines. The placebo is replaced by another vaccine or the same one in a different form so that the study becomes one of a comparison of two vaccines, not a comparison of the health of the vaccinated child with that of an unvaccinated. Tests also are only conducted on children who are healthy; thus roughly 60% of the general population of infants and children is not accepted into vaccine studies, yet the 'tested' vaccine is always given to this population as well as to the healthy.

Tests on vaccines are conducted by the pharmaceutical company who manufactures them – and thus often only the best results are reported, including on the company's package inserts. For example, the package insert for ActHib, (a vaccine for haemophilus influenzae (Hib), thought to cause meningitis) states:

"In a randomized, double-blind US clinical trial ActHIB was given concomitantly with DTP to more than 5,000 infants and Hepatitis B vaccine was given with DTP to a similar number. In this large study, deaths due to sudden infant death syndrome (SIDS) and other causes were observed but were not different in the two groups.

"In the first 48 hours following immunization, two definite and three possible seizures were observed after ActHIB and DTP in comparison with none after Hepatitis B vaccine and DTP alone. (Refer to product insert for AvP DTP). Other adverse reactions reported with administration of other Haemophilus b conjugate vaccines include urticaria, seizures, hives, renal failure and Guillain-Barre syndrome (GBS). A cause and effect relationship among any of these events and the vaccination has not been established."

In summary, Group A received Hib and DTP, the highly reactive vaccine for whooping cough that is no longer on the market in the US, and Group B received Hepatitis B and DTP. Vaccine reactions were then compared between the two groups. Both groups reported SIDS and seizures but these seem to be attributed to DTP as this had been previously reported for this vaccine. None of the other adverse reactions that "coincidentally" arose in these previously health infants during this trial were said to be causally related to the vaccine. Based on this information ActHib was judged safe and suitable for administration to practically all children, healthy or not.

---

[40] O'Shea, T. *The Sanctity of Human Blood: Vaccination I$ not Immunization.* Two Trees, San Jose, California, 2004

Jock Doubleday, director of the California's non-profit corporation, Natural Woman, Natural Man, Inc., offered a reward of $20,000 to any health professional who would publicly drink a mixture of standard vaccine additives in the same amount that a six-year old child is recommended to receive under the year-2005 guidelines of the U.S. Centers for Disease Control. On August 1, 2006, the reward was increased to $75,000. It was stated that the mixture will not contain viruses or bacteria dead or alive, but will contain standard vaccine additive ingredients in their usual forms and proportions.

The mixture will include, but will not be limited to, the following ingredients: thimerosal (a mercury derivative), ethylene glycol (antifreeze), phenol (a disinfectant dye), benzethonium chloride (a disinfectant), formaldehyde (a preservative and disinfectant), and aluminium microscopic needle-like crystals. The mixture will be body weight calibrated.

There have been no contenders for this reward, so...it was decided that, as of June 1, 2007, the $75,000 offer will increase to $80,000 and, as of July 1, 2007, the offer will increase to $85,000, as of August 1, 2007, the offer will increase to $90,000; as of September 1, 2007, the offer will increase to $95,000; as of October 1, 2007, the offer will increase to $100,000; as of November 1, 2007, the offer will increase to $105,000; as of December 1, 2007, the offer will increase to $110,000;as of January 1, 2008, the offer will increase to $115,000 . . . etc.

The offer will increase $5,000 per month, in perpetuity, until an M.D. or pharmaceutical company CEO, or anyone on vaccine regulatory committees, agrees to drink a body-weight calibrated dose of the poisonous vaccine additives that are routinely injected into children in the name of health. This offer, dated April 25, 2007, has no expiration date unless superseded by a similar offer of higher remuneration.

Chapter 5

Opinions About Jenner

Was Jenner's work accepted by everyone? No, there were anti-vaccinationists from the beginning. But Dr. Howard Haggard wrote in *Devils, Drugs and Doctors*, "The society of anti-vaccinationists was founded in the year that Jenner published his work and still continues actively. Its recruits come from that large class of persons who mistake fanatical opposition for intelligent criticism."[41] Three of the "fanatical and unintelligent" physicians of whom Haggard writes and who left writings behind are:

Walter Hadwen, J.P., M.D., L.R.C.P., M.R.C.S., L.S.A., (Gold Medalist in Medicine and Surgery). A verbatim report of his views on vaccination and his address at an assembly in Gloucester on January 25, 1896 still exists.[42]

Dr. Charles Creighton, one of the most lauded and important physicians of his time until he published *Natural History of Cowpox and Vaccinal Syphilis* in 1887 and publicly denounced vaccination. Because of his opposition he was ostracized by the medical community.

E.M. Crookshank, Professor of Comparative Pathology in King's College, London, published *History and Pathology of Vaccination* in 1889.

In this 'interview' with Dr. Hadwen, the dialogue has been extracted from the verbatim report of his address to the people of Gloucester.

$*$ $*$ $*$

Dr. Hadwen is a portly, white-whiskered gentleman with twinkly brown eyes. We are seated on studded, leather chairs in his London club. I, as a woman, have only been allowed in as a mark of respect for him but we have been hastily shepherded into a side room, not into the main lounge.

JC. Dr. Hadwen, I am sorry I missed your address on January 25. I hear that there was a large and enthusiastic audience. I am interested in your views of Edward Jenner and vaccination.

---

[41] Haggard, Howard. *Devils, Drugs and Doctors*. Harper, 1929. Pocket Book Edition 1946, p. 241

[42] http://whale.to/m/hadwen9.html

WH. You ask me about vaccination? As a medical man, I look upon vaccination as an insult to common sense, as superstitious in its origins, unscientific in theory and practice, and useless and dangerous in character.

JC. Those are strong words.

WH. The whole thing was a superstition of the Gloucestershire dairymaids years before Jenner was born and the very experiment, so-called, that he performed was 20 years earlier performed by an old farmer named Benjamin Jesty.

JC. So it wasn't true that a dose of cowpox prevented smallpox?

WH. When he first heard the story of the cowpox legend he began to mention it at the meetings of the medico-convivial society, where the old doctors of the day met to smoke their pipes, drink their glasses of grog, and talk over their cases. But he no sooner mentioned it than they laughed at it. The cow doctors could have told him of hundreds of cases where smallpox had followed cowpox.

Jenner got cases of those who had cowpox years before and had never had smallpox, as if everybody is bound to have the smallpox. Then he took some worn-out paupers, over 60 years of age, who had had the cowpox years and years before and inoculated them with smallpox to see if it would take. He found they did not take, because as people get advanced in life they are more or less proof against it. He took care in his paper never to mention the cases of people who had cowpox and had smallpox afterwards.

JC. Were there many cases of smallpox in the countryside? I thought that smallpox occurred in overcrowded, unhygienic conditions not usually found in the country?

WH. The period in which Jenner lived was undoubtedly a very filthy period. It was a time when, to take London for instance, the streets were nothing but a mass of cobble stones, the roads were so narrow that the people could almost shake hands across the street, and as for fresh air, they scarcely knew anything about it, for locomotion such as we have today was unknown.

Sanitary arrangements were altogether absent. They obtained their water from conduits and wells in the neighbourhood. Water closets there were none, and no drainage system existed. It was in London especially that smallpox abounded. Bodies were buried in Old St. Paul's Churchyard in Covent Garden only a foot below the soil, and people had to get up in the middle of the night and burn frankincense to keep off the stench. I say that smallpox is a filth disease and that if we get rid of the filth we shall get rid of the disease.

JC. Nevertheless, England made vaccination compulsory in 1853; why was that?

WH. The very moment you take a medical prescription and you incorporate it in an Act of Parliament, and you enforce it against the wills and conscience of intelligent people by fines, distraints and imprisonments, it passes beyond being a purely medical question – and becomes essentially a social and political one.

I may relate to you an amusing incident. A school inspector went to one of the schools the other day and asked this question of the class, 'Why was Moses hidden by his mother in the bulrushes?' A little fellow put up his hand and replied, 'Please sir, she did not want him vaccinated.'

(Laughter).

WH. *I also declare that when a person is ill, the doctor is justified in doing all he possibly can for his patient; but when a person is well he has no right whatever to interfere with the normal functions of the human body as he does when he introduces disease, especially the disease of an inferior animal.*

JC. *Is there any evidence at all that cowpox vaccination prevented smallpox?*

WH. *I will give you one or two statistics with regard to Leicester. In 1868–72 when 98% were vaccinated the mortality of children under one year was 107 per thousand. From 1888–9, when only 2% were vaccinated, the general mortality of children improved markedly to 63 per thousand.*

The vaccinationists say, 'Look at Prussia, and the way vaccination has stamped out smallpox there." Very well, we will look at Prussia, which, I may say has kept better vaccination records than any other country in Europe, except, perhaps Sweden. In 1834, which is twenty years before England adopted the Compulsory Vaccination Act, so severe was the Act in Prussia that, in addition to primary vaccination, every child had to be vaccinated over again when starting school life; he had to be re-vaccinated on going from college to college; and re-vaccinated again when he entered the Army, which meant every healthy male out of the whole of Prussia. And so severe was the Act that if any man refused to be vaccinated he was ordered to be held down and vaccinated by force; and so thoroughly was it done that he was vaccinated in ten places on each arm.

In 1871–2, thirty-five years after Prussia's Compulsory Vaccination Act, came the terrible epidemic which swept all over Europe. It came to Prussia, and what was the result? In that year smallpox carried off no less than 124,978 of her vaccinated and re-vaccinated citizens!

This roused Prussia, and she began to look about her; she saw the cause and determined to remedy it. She brought good water into her cities, purified her river Spree, introduced a complete drainage system throughout the country; and away fled the smallpox, like the Philistines before the Children of Israel. Sanitation did for Prussia what 35 years of compulsory vaccination was unable to accomplish. At the present time in Prussia smallpox is almost extinct.

JC. *With all this evidence, why do you suppose the medical men accepted it?*

WH. *In the first place science was then at a very low ebb. And the majority of doctors had never heard of or seen cowpox. When Jenner came forward with the letters F.R.S. and M.D. after his name, with all the impudence of a charlatan saying, 'Such is the singular character of my discovery that a person who is once inoculated with cowpox is for ever afterwards secure against smallpox,' the whole of the profession was arrested by the deliberate statement made, and they all bowed down before the golden calf which Nebuchadnezzar the king had set up.*

Another reason was that inoculation had turned out to be a failure. So when Jenner came forward and said, 'Here's a mild kind of smallpox; it's not infectious; it is certain to stop the smallpox,' why the doctors at once fell in with it and received it with open arms.

Another reason was that Jenner gave a scientific air to the whole thing by calling cowpox Variolae Vacciae. He may as well have called it diphtheria of the cow, for all the analogy it bore.

JC. I understand that people who received cowpox vaccination could be infected with other diseases. For example, James Phipps suffered from tuberculosis and indeed, Jenner's own son died of tuberculosis at age twenty."

WH. It is a very strange thing that up to 1853, when the Compulsory Vaccination Act was passed, the annual deaths from syphilis of children under one year old did not exceed 389; the very next year the number had jumped to nearly double, to 591; and syphilis in infants under one year of age has gone on increasing every year since until 1883, when the number of deaths reached 1,183. It has increased four-fold in infants since the passing of the Act and yet in adults it has remained almost stationary. Surely this speaks for itself.

*   *   *

I didn't want to tell him that over 100 years later people would venerate Jenner as the saviour of mankind from smallpox, nor that increased hygiene was not accompanied by an increase in awareness or of intelligence in the medical profession.

I have always been fascinated by the history of medicine, including nursing. As a student nurse I imagined myself working alongside Florence Nightingale in Crimea. From all accounts she had an acid tongue but, despite the constant rebukes I received from her in my imaginary ward, I was always inspired by the grateful eyes that peered at me from bandaged heads. Cleanliness, fresh air and good food were Florence's recipe for recovery and as a consequence we scrubbed until our hands were red and raw, we opened all available windows and we learned to cook nutritious broths for our men.

I own a battered paperback copy of Haggard's, *Devils, Drugs and Doctors*, first published in 1929. It cost me 42 cents. One can hope that most of Haggard's work is more accurate than his statements about vaccination. He says, "Queen Mary II of England died of smallpox in 1694. In the century following her death 60 million persons in Europe died of smallpox." The population of Europe was 130 million in 1762 and 175 million in 1800. The death rate from smallpox in that period was 18.5%. If 60 million deaths occurred with an 18.5% death rate then it would require 319,148,936 cases of smallpox in Europe and that would be 144,148,936 more cases of smallpox than there were people living in Europe at the close of the 18th century.[43]

One historical character I am fond of is Dr. Semmelweis, 1818–1865, who worked in the maternity hospital in Vienna. This hospital had two divisions: one for training medical students and the other for pupil midwives. In the first division, deaths averaged 99 per 1000 births; in the second, 33 per 1000 births. After considerable thought and inquiry, Semmelweis realised that medical students carried infection as they came straight from doing post-mortems to examining pre-

---

[43] Hale, A.R. *The Medical Voodoo*. Gotham House, New York, 1935

and post-natal women. He made them wash their hands in a solution of chloride of lime before touching the women. In the next 7 months the deaths fell to 12 per 1000.[44]

Was Semmelweis's discovery received with acclaim and gratitude? Absolutely not; he was greeted with hostility and official disdain. As they do today, the medical profession ignored the statistical evidence in favour of established practice.

Another character unjustly maligned was Dr. Charles Creighton, 1847-1927. Creighton was well-known and his book, *History of Epidemics in Great Britain*, was considered one of the greatest medical works ever written by one man. As a distinguished physician he was asked to write an article on the benefits of vaccination for the 1888 edition of the *Encyclopaedia Britannica*.[45] No one imagined that he would critically research the subject before writing. But he did and he was unable to come up with any actual benefits, much to the chagrin of the publishers and vaccine promoters.

In reference to the relationship between cow-pox and small-pox, Creighton wrote, "Jenner's originality consisted in boldly designating cow-pox as variolae vaccinae or smallpox of the cow, and in tracing cowpox itself back to the grease of horse's hocks. The latter contention was at length set aside by practical men as a crude fancy; the former designation is just as arbitrary and untenable. It was elaborately shown by Pearson in 1802, and has often been confirmed by subsequent writers, that the vesicle of inoculated cow-pox, even while it remains a vesicle, is quite unlike a single pustule of smallpox." (A vesicle is a blister filled with clear fluid in contrast to a pustule, a blister filled with pus.)

Creighton summarizes Jenner's work thus: "Jenner's originality in starting vaccination in practice is for the most part misunderstood. When he published his Inquiry in June 1798, he had twice succeeded in raising vaccine vesicles by experiment – the first time in June 1796 with matter from a milker's accidental sore, and the second time in March 1798 with matter direct from the cow. The first experiment was not carried beyond one remove from the cow; the second was carried to the fifth remove, when the succession failed. A third experiment, in the summer of 1798, failed from the outset; and his fourth and last experiment, in November – December 1798, led to nothing but extensive phagedenic (spreading) ulceration in two cases out of six vaccinated."

He goes on to describe five types of vaccination risk and includes the death rates in the vaccinated versus the unvaccinated. He then discusses the utility to the individual. "Do the vaccinated escape in an epidemic? Or, if they do not escape an attack of smallpox, do they escape death from it? In answer to the first question, apart from the familiar negative experience of everyone, we have the statistics of smallpox hospitals, which relate to the poorer class and probably do full justice to the fact of non-vaccination, inasmuch as the unvaccinated residue is mostly to be

---

[44] Haggard, p.84
[45] Creighton, C. Vaccination. *Encyclopaedia Brittanica*, Ninth Edition, 1875-1889, www.whale.to/creighton4.html

found in those slums and tenements of the poor where smallpox (now as always) is apt to linger. At the Eastern Metropolitan Hospital from its opening early in 1871 to the end of 1878 there were 6533 admissions for smallpox, of which 4283 had vaccination marks, 793 had no marks although vaccinated, and 1477 were unvaccinated giving a proportion of 0.29 unvaccinated." In other words of the 6533 cases of smallpox admitted to one hospital over a seven-year period, 71% had been vaccinated.

Creighton answers the second question about death rates with a series of tables. "In pre-vaccination times the death rate (18.8%) was almost the same as it is now in the vaccinated and unvaccinated together."

Needless to say his article was left out of the next edition of the encyclopaedia and was replaced by a piece about glycerinated calf lymph as a vaccine, written by one of its promoters.

In 1889 Creighton expressed his views in a more popular form in *Jenner & Vaccination*, published by Cassell & Co. In it he wrote, "The public at large cannot believe that a great profession should have been so perseveringly in the wrong. The profession as a whole has been committed before now to erroneous doctrines and injurious practices, which have been upheld by its solid authority for generations. It is difficult to conceive what will be the excuse made for a century of cowpoxing; but it cannot be doubted that the practice will appear in as absurd a light to the common sense of the twentieth century as bloodletting now does to us."[46]

Dr. Creighton died in poverty on July 18th, 1927. An obituary appeared in *The Lancet* written by Professor William Bulloch, which included the following statements:

"By the death of Charles Creighton, England has lost her most learned medical scholar of the nineteenth century, although it cannot be forgotten that some of his opinions were the subject of such criticism that he ceased to be felt as a power in the medical world."

Bulloch goes on: "The real tragedy of Creighton's life was connected with his views on cowpox and vaccination. His article in the ninth edition of *Encyclopaedia Brittanica* literally sealed his fate... The issue between Creighton and general professional opinion on vaccination was not thrashed out there and then as it ought to have been. It was deemed more expedient to drop Creighton into oblivion, and if he was ever referred to at all it was only as 'Creighton the Anti-Vaccinator.' All his other work was forgotten in the debacle, and he was a doomed man. In the opinion of many he was harshly treated by the world for holding views that did not conform to standard."[47]

Do we treat people with non-conformist views any differently today? I don't think so. And today we have the influence of the giant pharmaceutical industry

---

[46] Swan, Joseph. *The Vaccination Problem*, 1936.
[47] Swan, J. "Dr. Creighton and Prof. Crookshank". Chapter 4, *The Vaccination Problem*, 1936.www.whale/to

which quashes non-conformists by removing their grants. The control currently exercised by the pharmaceutical industry will be discussed later as it has a right to its own chapter.

> *Dear Dr. Creighton: You won't believe this but it is now the twenty-first century and people still believe that the cowpox virus prevents smallpox! Furthermore, they are sure that smallpox has been eradicated by the vaccine.*
> *Don't get dizzy revolving in your grave.*

The third in the trio of "fanatical and unintelligent" physicians, Dr. E. M. Crookshank, Professor of Comparative Pathology in King's College, London, was investigating an outbreak of cowpox in Wiltshire for the Agricultural Department. He became so impressed with the lack of knowledge about cowpox in medical practitioners that he undertook his own investigation and published, in 1889, a two-volume work entitled *History and Pathology of Vaccination*. (London: H. K. Lewis.) Joseph Swan provides a few extracts from Crookshank's book. [48]

"Unfortunately, a belief in the efficacy of vaccination has been so enforced in the education of the medical practitioner, that it is hardly probable that the futility of the practice will be generally acknowledged in our generation, though nothing would be more redound to the credit of the profession and give evidence of the advance made in pathology and sanitary science."

Given the prestige and authority of Drs. Creighton and Crookshank, it is astonishing that vaccination did not meet its timely end there and then. Swan suggests that they were academics, not in general practice, and were, therefore, confronted with the enormous dead weight of the professional interests of the government medical officials and general practitioners. For example, *The Lancet* (13th April, 1889) stated, "It is about as rational to investigate the merits and value of vaccination as a security against smallpox as it would be to question the utility of life-boats, or Davy lamps, or fire brigades."

---

[48] Swan, Joseph. *The Vaccination Problem.* 1936

Chapter 6

Smallpox

Last week I received one of those E mails from a well-meaning friend that warned me about a virus that would make my computer drop dead or spread destruction throughout my files or send lewd messages to everyone in my address book. As I normally do in such cases, I referred to the "hoaxbusters" website and sure enough, there was a copy of the warning I had received. It had been circulating for three years.

How do we know when we are the victim of a hoax? Who do we believe? Many people put their faith in the words of a few elite who are generally considered to possess superior knowledge. How many people thought they had found the truth in Waco or Jonestown, for example? I have always been wary of charismatic leaders as I am not naturally a follower and I yawn when yet another one is found to be a sexual predator or has absconded with the funds.

There are many people who hate to be confused by facts, especially when those facts fly in the face of their cherished beliefs. I have always loved the Hans Christian Andersen story, *The Emperor's New Clothes*. I want to be the child who points to the king and shouts, "The king is as naked as the day that he was born" and force people to correct their impaired vision.

The history of smallpox is worth studying because it was this disease that started vaccine mythology. The word 'pox' is the plural form of 'pocke' (pocke meaning sac). Smallpox leaves small indentations, pocks, all over the body but particularly over the face. The name 'smallpox", which first occurs in Holinshead's *Chronicles* from 1571, was given to this disease to distinguish it from syphilis, the 'great pox'.

Michael Nightingale, a practitioner of Traditional Chinese Medicine, writes: "It is a matter of pure speculation as to when the condition first appeared, but it is unlikely to have done so prior to man's establishment of large townships coupled with poor nutrition, overcrowding, lack of sanitation and inadequate hygiene. Keeping people, such as slaves and prisoners, in disgusting and sub-human conditions may have been the necessary ingredient for the establishment of the virus but there is virtually no doubt that the aforementioned adverse conditions were responsible for the epidemics of smallpox as well as for its endemic nature in certain areas until its recent demise. It was recorded in Chinese history and was certainly prevalent in the west by the sixteenth century."[49]

Claims that vaccination is responsible for the decline in smallpox are facile. The incontrovertible fact is that smallpox declined with declining vaccination rates. In answer to a parliamentary question by the British Minister of Health on July 16th, 1923, a written list of figures of vaccinations and deaths from 1872 – 1921 was presented.[50] I have averaged the figures here into 10 year periods.

Years	Vaccinations per 100 births	Deaths from Smallpox	Deaths from Smallpox per 100,000 population	Deaths from cowpox and other effects of vaccination
1872-1881	85.5	1999	15.2	344
1882-1891	82.2	923	34.1	497
1892–1901	68.0	436	1.4	366
1902–1911	67.4	395	1.2	17.7
1912–1921	43.5	12	0.1	83

You can see from these figures that as compliance with vaccination went down so did the death rate – quite the opposite to what the medical establishment now tells us.

The report of Dr. William Farr, Compiler of Statistics of the Registrar General of London states: "Smallpox attained its maximum mortality after vaccination was introduced. The mean annual mortality for 10,000 population from 1850 to 1869 was at the rate of 2.04, whereas after compulsory vaccination in 1871 the death rate was 10.24. In 1872 the death rate was 8.33 and this after the most laudable efforts to extend vaccination by legislative enactments."[51]

By 1919, England and Wales had become one of the least vaccinated countries and had only 28 deaths from smallpox out of a population of 37.8 million people.[52] According to official figures of the Registrar General of England, 109 children under five years in England and Wales died of smallpox between 1910 and 1933. In that same period 270 died from vaccination.[53] Between 1934 and

---

[49] Nightingale, M. Smallpox: Why all the Fuss? www.whale.to/vaccines/smallpox4.html

[50] Hadwen, Walter. The Fraud of Vaccination. *Truth*, January 3, 1923

[51] McBean, E. *The Poisoned Needle*. Health Research, Pomeroy. WA, 1993

[52] Krasner, G. The Dangers of Vaccination. www.naturodoc.com

[53] Sinclair, I. *Vaccination: The "Hidden" Facts*, Australia, 1992

1961 not one smallpox death was recorded but 115 children under five years died from smallpox vaccination.[54]

Apart from killing people the literature abounds with examples of the failure of smallpox vaccination to prevent the disease.

One of the worst smallpox epidemics took place in England between 1870 and 1872, nearly two decades after compulsory vaccination was introduced. Leicester, with nearly 200,000 inhabitants, boasted a 95% vaccination record but it suffered more deaths than less-vaccinated London. Faced with this obvious evidence of the uselessness of vaccination, Leicester's citizens rejected the program in favour of cleaning up the city. Under the leadership of James Briggs, Town Councillor and Sanitary Inspector, clean streets, clean markets and dairies, efficient garbage removal, sanitary housing and pure water supply replaced vaccination scars.[55] In 1892-3 Leicester had 19.3 cases of smallpox per 10,000 population; while similar-sized Warrington, with 99.2% vaccinated, had 123.3 cases per 10,000 – over six times as many.[56]

In Japan, in 1885, 13 years after compulsory vaccination, a law was passed requiring re-vaccination every seven years. From 1886 to 1892 a total of 25,474,370 revaccinations were recorded. Yet during this same period, Japan had 156,175 cases of smallpox with 38,979 deaths, a case mortality of nearly 25 percent. Slow learners, the government passed another act requiring every resident to be vaccinated and re-vaccinated every 5 years. Between 1889–1908, the case mortality was 30 percent. Prior to vaccination the case mortality was about 10 percent.[57]

During a ruthless campaign by the US in the Philippines in 1905, the native population were forcibly vaccinated several times. In 1918–1919, with over 95% of the population vaccinated, the worst epidemic the Philippines had ever known occurred. In the *Congressional Record* of December 21, 1937, William Howard Hay, MD, said, "The Philippines suffered the worst attack of smallpox, the worst epidemic three times over, that had ever occurred in the history of the islands and it was almost three times as fatal. The death rate ran as high as 60% in certain areas where formerly it had been 10-15%."[58]

The same Dr. Hay addressed the Medical Freedom Society regarding the Lemke Bill to abolish compulsory vaccination. He stated, "I have thought many times of all the insane things we have advocated in medicine, that one of the most insane was to insist on the vaccination of children, or anybody else, for the prevention of smallpox when, as a matter of fact, we are never able to prove that vaccination saved one man from smallpox.

"It is nonsense to think that you can inject pus – and it is usually from the pustule end of the dead smallpox victim – it is unthinkable that you can inject that

---

[54] Ransom, S. Lies, Damn Lies and Statistics. www.campaignfortruth.com
[55] Hale, AR. *The Medical Voodoo*. Gotham House Inc. 1935
[56] Ransom, S. Lies, Damn Lies and Statistics, campaignfortruth.com, 2003
[57] Sinclair, Ian. *Vaccination: The Hidden Facts*. Australia, 1992
[58] Ibid.

into a little child and in any way improve its health. What is true of vaccination is exactly as true of all forms of serum immunization, so called, if we could by any means build up a natural resistance to disease through these artificial means, I would applaud it to the echo, but we can't do it."[59]

Objections to smallpox vaccination continued into the twentieth century. Dr. R. P. Garrow published an article in a January 1928 issue of the *British Medical Journal* showing that the fatality rate among the vaccinated smallpox cases over 15 years of age in England and Wales in 1923 and 1926 was higher than among the unvaccinated. The article provoked a number of letters including one from Dr. L. A. Parry. He raised a number of questions:

1.   How is it that smallpox is five times as likely to be fatal in the vaccinated as in the unvaccinated?

2.   How is it that, as the percentage of people vaccinated has steadily fallen (from 85% in 1870 to about 40% in 1925), the number of people attacked with variola has declined *pari passu* and the case mortality has progressively lessened? The years of least vaccination have been the years of least smallpox and of least mortality.

3.   How is that in some of our best vaccinated towns – for example Bombay and Calcutta – smallpox is rife, whilst in some of our worst vaccinated towns, such as Leicester, it is almost unknown?

4.   How is it that something like 80% of the cases admitted into the Metropolitan Asylum Board smallpox hospitals have been vaccinated whilst only 20% have not been vaccinated?

5.   How is it that in Germany, the best vaccinated country in the world, there are more deaths in proportion to the population than in England -- for example, in 1919, 28 deaths in England, 707 in Germany; in 1920, 30 deaths in England, 354 in Germany. In Germany, in 1919 there were 5,012 cases of smallpox with 707 deaths; in England in 1925 there were 5,363 cases of smallpox with 6 deaths. What is the explanation?

6.   Is it possible to explain the lessened incidence and fatality of smallpox on the same grounds as the lessened incidence and fatality of other infectious fevers – namely, as due to improved hygiene and administrative control?

Dr. Parry finished his letter with: "These are just a few points in connection with the subject which are puzzling me, and to which I want answers. I am in doubt, and I want to know the truth. Will some of the experts help me?"

The experts represented by the journal commented: "We think Dr. Parry, in his desire for enlightenment, would have been wiser not to introduce assumptions of fact into the framework of his questions."[60]

---

[59] Ibid.

[60] Scheibner, V. *Vaccination: 100 Years of Orthodox Research Shows that Vaccination Represents a Medical Assault on the Immune System.* New Atlantean Press, 1993

Perhaps the best source for understanding the evolution of vaccination until the early twentieth century is Annie Riley Hale's *The Medical Voodoo* published in New York in 1935. A medical historian, Hale gives numerous fascinating references and quotations from medical literature and from American papers and journals. She deals mainly with smallpox vaccination because the myriad vaccines of today had, of course, not been developed.

I have come to realise that pointing out the obvious does not elicit change, either in thinking or in how things are done. My first lesson was when I was a nineteen-year old student nurse on my first night duty. We worked from 9PM until 8AM on large, open wards that were designed by Florence Nightingale so that each of the 34 patients was surrounded by the requisite number of cubic feet of air.

In the morning, before the day staff came on duty, two student nurses were expected to serve tea, do a bedpan or bottle round, administer medicines and injections, take TPRs (temperature, pulse, respirations), change dressings, do treatments such as enemas or catheterizations, collect specimens, AND bed-bath the four sickest patients. Never mind handling incontinence, emergencies or deaths.

In order to accomplish this overwhelming work list, we bed-bathed the sick patients when they woke up in the night or between 5AM and 6AM, leaving the rest of the tasks to be done between 6 and 8 AM, that is, in two hours. Then came the edict from Matron's Office – we were not to bath any patient before 6 AM.

Right, I thought, they obviously don't understand what we have to do. So I wrote out all the tasks and a conservative estimate of how long each took. The total time exceeded three hours and that was without any unexpected events or emergencies.

I trotted off to Matron's Office in the middle of the night when I knew the Night Sisters would be there and presented them with my list. To my surprise it was not received with enlightenment and cries of wonder; the word "impertinence" figured prominently and I was told to go back to my ward and get on with it.

This and other experiences working as an educational consultant in a medical school assures me that factual data do nothing to change people's minds. The trouble is, I don't know what does.

I find the following two letters particularly interesting.[61]

July, 1931
Dear George Bernard Shaw:
A few years ago I believe you stated that you were opposed to vaccination. It has been said that great men frequently change their minds, and I should like to ask whether you still condemn vaccination?

Will you forgive me if I ask whether you have ever been successfully vaccinated? The subject of vaccination is one that interests millions of persons,

---

[61] Hale, A.R. *The Medical Voodoo*. Gotham House, Inc. 1935

and is my excuse for asking these personal questions. With best wishes for a long, healthy life, I am,

   Yours very truly,
   Chas. F. Pabst, M.D.
   And the reply came:
   London, July 19, 1931
   Dr. Pabst:
   I was vaccinated in infancy and had 'good marks' of it. In the great epidemic of 1881 (I was born in 1856) I caught smallpox. During the last considerable epidemic at the turn of the century, I was a member of the Health Committee of London Borough Council, and I learned how the credit of vaccination is kept up statistically by diagnosing all the re-vaccinated cases as pustular eczema, varioloid, or what-not – except smallpox. I discovered a suppressed report of the Metropolitan Asylums Board on a set of re-vaccinations which had produced extraordinarily disastrous results. Meanwhile I had studied the literature and statistics of the subject. I even induced a celebrated bacteriologist to read Jenner. I have no doubt whatever that vaccination is an unscientific abomination and should be made a criminal practice.
   G. Bernard Shaw

   The idea of re-naming a disease to suit the records is not new. Hadwen, the man I "interviewed", also said in his address that in 1886, although there were 275 cases of smallpox, only one vaccinated child died. In addition, 93 children died of chicken pox. Chicken pox? The mildest of childhood diseases.

   The re-naming practice continues today. In 1967 the World Health Organization (WHO) began a campaign to eradicate smallpox, a campaign that was carefully monitored. In 1979 Arita and Breman wrote "Interhuman transmission of smallpox, which continued for more than 3000 years, appears to have come to an end on 26 October 1977, when the world's last known case developed his rash in Merca, Somalia."[62]

   The disease was officially declared eradicated on May 8, 1980. Part of the statement was, "… since there is no human carrier state of epidemiological importance and **no recognised animal reservoir of the disease**, the absence of clinically apparent cases in man may be assumed to signify the absence of a naturally occurring smallpox." (My emphasis).

   No animal reservoir? Scheibner follows a discussion about the inability to distinguish between various pox viruses – monkeypox, whitepox, camelpox – and the smallpox virus in the laboratory. These pox-family viruses have been known for many years but the public has been reassured that they have nothing to do with smallpox and that the human species is safe.

---

[62] Scheibner, V. *Vaccination: 100 Years of Orthodox Research Shows that Vaccination Represents a Medical Assault on the Immune System.* New Atlantean Press, 1993

Since 1970, pox viruses found in captive monkeys have been isolated in humans and a new disease, first known as 'monkeypox' and now 'human monkeypox', has materialised. So what is the difference between smallpox and monkeypox? A 1977 *Lancet* article informs us that, "Human monkeypox is a systemic exanthema, resembling smallpox, that occurs as a sporadic zoonosis in rural rainforest villages of western and central Africa. The disease is caused by an orthopoxvirus, which is transmitted to human beings by handling infected animals; serosurveys have implicated squirrels ... as the probable reservoir. Secondary human-to-human spread by aerosol or direct contact accounts for about 28% of cases."[63]

'Exanthema' means a rash and in this case it <u>resembles</u> smallpox. Apparently this look-alike smallpox is quite infectious since there were 42 cases, including 3 deaths, reported in a village with only 346 inhabitants.[64]

The difference between the smallpox virus and the human monkeypox virus is a difference in protein structure. As health authorities have never worried about the difference between cowpox virus and smallpox virus, why should they be concerned now? Concerned enough, that is, to say that monkeypox is not smallpox. They can't have it both ways: saying the cowpox virus prevents smallpox but then denying that the monkeypox virus can cause smallpox. Clinically, the diseases are the same. Even the CDC on its webpage admits that the signs and symptoms of monkeypox are like those of smallpox. They go on to say that the death rate in Africa is 1-10% but the risk would be lower in the US because of better nutrition and hygiene. It is odd that they've never acknowledged the role of nutrition and hygiene before – but that was when they were advocating vaccination.

One benefit that has resulted from the declaration that smallpox has been eradicated is that vaccination is no longer mandatory or advocated. So that is something to be thankful for.

CHOLERA

I have a home video of my children demonstrating to their South African cousins that the water in a flushing toilet in the northern hemisphere swirls in the opposite direction to theirs. Although it is amusing it makes me reflect on how readily we accept flush toilets, garbage pickup and clean water. Because of systems that we take for granted, it is hard to imagine the conditions in Britain in the nineteenth century. Charles Dickens describes some in *Bleak House* and in *Nicholas Nickleby* but an article by Mayhew, published in the London *Morning*

---

[63] Gaublomme K. Has smallpox really disappeared from the earth? www.whale/to

[64] Schreibner V. *Vaccination: 100 Years of Orthodox Research Shows that Vaccination Represents a Medical Assault on the Immune System*. New Atlantean Press, 1993

Chronicle in 1849, painted an even more shocking picture by simply describing what he witnessed.[65]

"We then journeyed on to London-street... In No.1 of this street the cholera first appeared seventeen years ago, and spread up it with fearful virulence; but this year it appeared at the opposite end, and ran down it with like severity. As we passed along the reeking banks of the sewer, the sun shone upon a narrow slip of the water. In the bright light it appeared the colour of strong green tea, and positively looked as solid as black marble in the shadow – indeed, it was more like watery mud than muddy water; and yet we were assured this was the only water the wretched inhabitants had to drink. As we gazed in horror at it, we saw a whole tier of doorless privies in the open road, common to men and women, built over it; we heard bucket after bucket of filth splash into it; and the limbs of the vagrant boys bathing in it seemed by pure force of contrast white as Parian marble. And yet, as we stood doubting the fearful statement, we saw a little child, from one of the galleries opposite, lower a tin can with a rope to fill a large bucket that stood beside her. In each of the balconies that hung over the stream the self-same tub was to be seen in which the inhabitants put the mucky liquid to stand, so that they may, after it rested for a day or two, skim the fluid from the solid particles of filth, pollution and disease. As the little thing dangled her tin cup as gently as possible into the stream, a bucket of night-soil was poured down from the next gallery."

(Night-soil is defined in the Oxford English Dictionary as "the excrementitious matter removed by night from cesspools etc.")

Vibrio cholerae is the bacterium that causes cholera. Normally harmless. it can wreak havoc in the small intestine when it injects a toxin that disrupts the body's water balance. The walls of the small intestine are lined with two types of cells: one that absorbs water and one that excretes it. In health there is a balance but the cholera toxin tricks the cells into expelling water, so much so that, in extreme cases, a victim can lose up to 30% of body weight in a few hours.

The liquid stool from cholera sufferers contains millions of *vibrio cholerae* and as they have to be ingested to reach another small intestine, it is imperative that even minute quantities of stool do not reach the water supply. Given the conditions described by Mayhew it is hardly surprising that in the cholera epidemic of 1848-1849, over 50,000 people died.[66]

I mention cholera because, in reading about vaccination, smallpox is so emphasised that it is easy to forget that other diseases took their toll in the same era. Until John Snow discovered the connection between water and sewage around 1854, cholera patients were treated with castor oil and blood letting. What surprises me is that no enterprising charlatan came forward with the notion of injecting night-soil under the skin. After all, that idea is no more farfetched than scraping pus into an incision. No, cholera was eliminated by providing clean water and building sewers. Vaccination was unnecessary. Leicester eliminated smallpox

---

[65] Johnson. S. *The Ghost Map*. Riverhead Books, 2006
[66] Ibid.

in the same way; nevertheless, a smallpox vaccination was still considered necessary.

I recently saw a TV documentary that showed African children scooping up muddy water in plastic buckets for the family's consumption. The West, however, still conducts vaccination campaigns rather than using this money to provide clean water and sewers. The question is, whose interests are being served by this practice?

Chapter 7

Childhood Diseases

There's an attitude in today's society that no child should ever get sick from an infectious disease; in Western society that is. Chronic diseases like asthma seem to be far more acceptable. For example, the *Electronic Telegraph*, January 11th, 2000 printed this piece:

LOUISE HAD MEASLES – NEEDLESSLY

Louise Bate is gazing listlessly from her mother's arms, showing little interest in her toys or her three-year old brother, William, playing on the floor. Aged nine months, she is recovering from a dose of measles that has left her drained of energy. Louise's mother Josie is indignant that Louise has fallen ill. "I feel very frustrated and sad that she got an illness that could have been avoided. Louise went from being a totally contented, happy, sleeping, well-feeding baby to the most miserable, distressed, sick child – and I know from my GP that she didn't have it badly. Measles can cause complications such as brain damage and hearing loss."

Clearly, Louise's mother does not know that the complications from a *measles vaccine* are possibly autism, meningitis, arthritis, brain damage and a defective muscular control that results in jerky movements.[67] If she was asked to balance these conditions against a few days of feeling "miserable and distressed" I wonder which she would choose.

Alternative practitioners like homeopaths believe the function of "childhood" diseases is to prime immature immune systems as a necessary condition for health. Reports of developmental leaps following chicken pox for example are common but are dismissed as subjective. After all, what do mothers know?

There are, however, studies to support these observations. *The Annals of Tropical Paediatrics* reports the case of a 5-year old girl with a bad case of psoriasis that resisted all treatment. When she came down with measles, the

---

[67] Null, G. *Vaccines: a Second Opinion*. www.garynull.com

measles rash replaced the psoriasis, which never reappeared. Another study showed that the prevalence of parasites is significantly lower in children who have had measles or influenza before the age of nine than in the control group.

People do not appreciate that *getting childhood diseases is the only way to acquire immunity against them,* and lifelong immunity in most cases. The term 'immunization' is a misnomer as vaccinations clearly do not confer long-lasting immunity or else there would be no need for 'booster' shots.

My grandmother's generation and indeed, my own, didn't expect kids to live without infectious disease, aches and injuries, for which they harboured tried and true home remedies. They would find it incomprehensible that this generation is willing to tolerate asthma, food allergies and autism instead of chicken pox.

Death rates from infectious diseases were dropping significantly by the beginning of the twentieth century. However, from 1911 to 1935 the four leading causes of death among those aged 1 to 14 were reported to be diphtheria, measles, scarlet fever and whooping cough.

Diphtheria

Early in my nurse training, when I was keen and eager to serve humanity, we were told how to perform an emergency tracheotomy. Such a procedure could save the life of someone with obstructed breathing, diphtheria being the most likely cause. We were to cut the skin of the throat, locate the windpipe – the trachea – slit it and insert a tube. The trachea is made of tough fibre and, we were warned, requires strength and a sharp knife to cut it. A handy tube is the inside of a ballpoint pen. This must be inserted quickly as the tracheal slit will close if not held open.

I mentally rehearsed the procedure so often that I would know exactly what to do when called upon.

Fingering the ballpoint pen in my pocket I am walking down a Leeds street when a woman rushes out of her mean dwelling. "Help me," she cries. "My baby is dying."

"Fear not," I yell and leap into the house. A toddler is gasping, his face blue, his limbs flaccid. "Quick. Get me a sharp knife," I order the distraught woman as I lift the unconscious child on to the only table.

"Be not alarmed, Madam," I say with knife poised. No, that won't do.

"Don't worry, luv," I say with knife poised. "Would you get me some soap, hot water and a towel."

While she is gone, I unscrew the ballpoint pen, extract the inner tube and empty out the ink. I quickly cut the skin of the child's throat. It hardly bleeds. The trachea is obvious. I slit it with a decisive thrust of the knife and insert the tube. There is a rushing noise. The child begins to breathe. His face turns pink.

"Oh, you have saved my baby," the mother cries when she returns with the towel. "How can I ever thank you?"

The heavenly host break into song. The mother gazes at me adoringly.

"It was nothing." I lower my eyes modestly.

"What is your name? I shall call my next child after you."

I can feel a halo surround my head.

*   *   *

I never did get to perform a tracheotomy, emergency or otherwise although I did nurse many people with them, none with diphtheria.

The name diphtheria is derived from the Greek, *diphthera*, meaning leather hide. Hippocrates described the disease in the 5th century BCE so it's been around for a long time. I suspect it was called leather hide because, in this bacterial respiratory disease, membranes form in the throat, particularly over the tonsils and the larynx.

Like whooping cough and tetanus, diphtheria is classified as a toxin-mediated disease because the bacterium itself does not cause the damage – this is from toxins produced by cells in response to the bacteria. Antitoxins were tried out in the 1930s but the protection was transient, lasting only 6-8 weeks. Furthermore, antitoxin was made in horses and caused severe reactions such as anaphylaxis and serum sickness.

"Four separate studies done in 1934, 1935 and 1937, found that Vitamin C had the power to neutralise, inactivate and render harmless diphtheria toxins."[68] Yet this important treatment is ignored. Could the reason be that vitamins are not patentable?

The USA recorded death rates from 1901.[69] In that year 48,839 people died from diphtheria, or about 40 per 100,000. In 1946 there were 467 deaths, or about 1.2 per 100,000. Over 45 years a fall from 48,839 down to 467? That seems like a significant drop. Yet it was in 1946 that the vaccine for diphtheria was introduced.

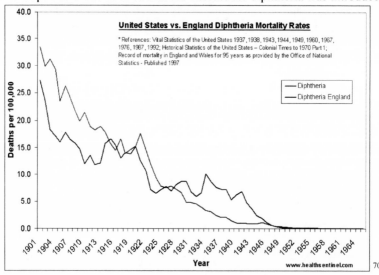

[68] Butler, Hilary. Diphtheria. www.alternative-doctor.com

[69] Alderson, M. International Mortality Statistics. *Facts on File, Inc.* 1981

[70] This and subsequent graphs in this chapter are from "Vaccines do not save us." www.childhealthsafety.wordpress.com/graphs/

Mendelsohn, a paediatrician, says, "Today your child has about as much chance of contracting diphtheria as she does of being bitten by a cobra. Yet millions of children are immunized against it with repeated injections at two, four, six, and eighteen months and then given a booster shot when they enter school. This, despite evidence from over more than a dozen years of rare outbreaks of the disease, that children who have been immunized fare no better than those who have not. For example, during a 1969 outbreak of diphtheria in Chicago the city board of health reported that four of the sixteen victims had been fully immunized against the disease and five others had received one or more doses of the vaccine."[71]

Measles
"Christopher Robin had wheezles and sneezles, they bundled him into his bed. They gave him what goes with a cold in the nose, and some more for a cold in the head. They wondered if wheezles could turn into measles, if sneezles could turn into mumps; they examined his chest for a rash, and the rest of his body for lumps."

I grew up on Christopher Robin. My favourite soft toy was Eeyore and neither he nor I would dream of treading on the lines in the street. I too, had wheezles that turned into measles. We all had measles as children. My mother's generation could recognise the spots and diagnose the disease without medical help. Any of my contemporaries I've asked know they had measles but they remember nothing of it. It was a non-event as measles is a mild self-limiting viral childhood disease that commonly resolves in a week. The symptoms are itching red spots, fatigue, and the fever that is a good sign of a healthy immune response. The treatment is to stay in bed, drink lots of non-sugared drinks and apply calamine lotion to the spots.

Today the Health Authorities have convinced everyone that encephalitis lurks under every measles bed if you have not had their measles shot and the media refer to measles as "deadly." However, Mendelsohn, [72] says: "Doctors maintain that the (MMR) inoculation is necessary to prevent measles encephalitis, which they say occurs about once in 1,000 cases. After decades of experience with measles, I question this statistic, and so do many other paediatricians. The incidence of 1/1,000 may be accurate for children who live in conditions of poverty and malnutrition, but in the middle-and upper-income brackets, if one excludes simple sleepiness from the measles itself, the incidence of true encephalitis is probably more like 1/10,900 or 1/100,000."

Mendelsohn's observation is supported by an international biostatistician, Michael Alderson, who says that, as there were 44 deaths from measles in the

---

[71] Mendelsohn, R. The Medical Time Bomb of Immunization Against Disease. www.whale.to/vaccines/mendelsophn.html

[72] Mendelsohn, R. *How to Raise a Healthy Child in Spite of your Doctor*, Random House, 1987

entire 5-year period from 1965-1970 in the US, this would be an incidence of less than 1 in 100,000 [73]

In the U.S. the death rate from measles was 13.3 per 100,000 in 1900, 0.2 in 1945 and zero in 1970. The single measles vaccine was introduced in 1963 but was pulled off the market in 1967 because it was causing a severe form of measles, which was presumed to be because the vaccinated children had come into contact with the natural virus.[74] Between 1971 and 1975, a four-year period, there were 17 deaths in the whole of the U.S.A. The combined Measles, Mumps and Rubella (MMR) vaccine was only introduced in 1978.

A study published in *Archives of Internal Medicine* (and there are few more prestigious journals than that) evaluated all U.S. and Canadian articles reporting measles outbreaks in schools. On average, 77% of all cases occurred in vaccinated individuals. The statistics just do not confirm that measles vaccine stops measles. A measles epidemic happened in three schools in the U.S.A despite everyone of the students, about 4,200 of them, being vaccinated, despite a vaccination density of 96%, meaning nearly everyone was vaccinated, Fife in Scotland still had measles epidemics in 1991 and 1992.[75]

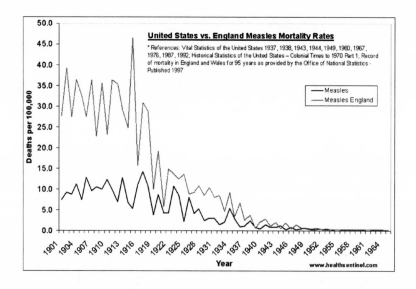

[73] O'Shea, T. *The Sanctity of Human Blood: Vaccination I$ not Immunization.* Two Trees, San Jose, California, 2004

[74] Miller, N. *Vaccine Safety Manual.* New Atlantean Press, 2008

[75] Carter, H. "Measles outbreak in Fife: which MMR policy." *Public Health*, January 1993

Scarlet Fever

I had scarlet fever when I was three and I spent some time in a 'fever' hospital. The only incident I remember was receiving two parcels. I was thrilled. I don't recall what was in them but I was told, presumably by a nurse, that I was only allowed one. I could choose one and she took the other away. The injustice rankles today. Such was the authoritarianism of that era; people in power who know what is best for everyone else.

The death rate for scarlet fever in the U.S. was about 14 per 100,000 in 1900 and fell to zero in 1951.

There is no vaccine for scarlet fever. "Scarlet fever was always every bit as fatal as diphtheria. That it declined in every way, both in incidence and in so-called virulence, as rapidly as did diphtheria and all without a vaccine or an anti-toxin, should have vital meaning for every truth seeker."[76]

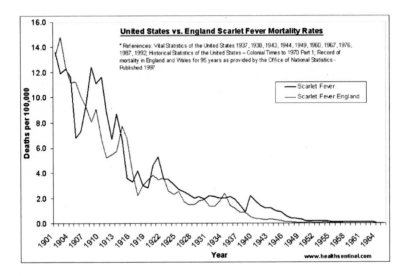

Whooping Cough

Pertussis is the medical name for whooping cough, a nasty bacterial disease that killed many infants in past centuries. With violent coughing, so deep that all air is expelled and a characteristic whooping sound caused by the desperate inhaling to refill the empty lungs. Like most other infectious diseases, whooping cough was found alongside poverty, malnutrition, unsafe water, poor hygiene, and overcrowding. Pertussis deaths fell from 12.2 per 100,000 in 1900 to 1.3 in 1945 in the U.S. The vaccine was introduced in 1946.

---

[76] Shelton, H. Why we have epidemics. Quoted in Sinclair.

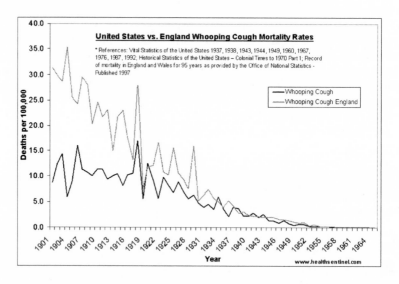

In an outbreak of pertussis in Nova Scotia in 1990, 93% of the affected children had received three or more vaccinations. In 1994, the *New England Journal of Medicine* published a study showing that pertussis vaccine "failed to give protection against the disease." More than 80% of the cases in a recent epidemic had received regular doses of vaccine.[77]

BBC News, July 7, 2006, reported "Whooping cough still widespread." University of Oxford researchers had studied 172 children and found whooping cough among them despite 85% being vaccinated. They suggested that GPs consider this diagnosis even where there is a history of vaccination. A spokesman for the UK Health Protection Agency said: "We're fully aware that protection from the vaccine wears off." As pertussis breaks out about every three to four years and as the vaccine seems to be ineffective, why give it at all?

In England and Wales there was a 90% decline in child *mortality* from the combined infectious diseases of diphtheria, measles, scarlet fever and pertussis in the period 1850 -1940.[78] In the US, an organization other than a health related one, the Metropolitan Life Insurance Company's 1948 report states, "… the combined death rate of diphtheria, measles, scarlet fever and whooping cough declined 95% among children ages 1-14 from 1911 to 1945 before the mass immunization programs started in the United States.[79]

Although scurvy is not classified as a childhood disease it is interesting to compare the deaths from scurvy with those above:

---

[77] Miller, NZ. *Immunisation: Theory vs. Reality*. New Atlantean Press, 1996
[78] Department of Health and Social Security, UK.
[79] O'Shea, T. *The Sanctity of Human Blood: Vaccination I$ not Immunization*. Two Trees, San Jose, California, 2004

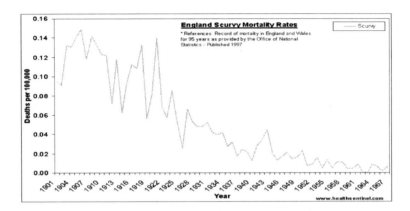

I turn to the Canadian authority on vaccines – Health Canada and its magazine article, *Vaccination: Myths and Facts.*[80]

The first "<u>Myth</u>" according to the article is "Diseases started to disappear before vaccines were introduced, because of better hygiene and sanitation."

No one is saying that diseases disappeared; they are saying the <u>death rates</u> declined, meaning that they are not deadly as Health Canada would have us believe.

The article then goes on with the <u>Fact</u>. "It's true that improved social and economic conditions have had an impact on our health. Better nutrition, antibiotics and other treatments, less crowded living conditions and lower birth rates have helped keep disease in check." *Note how they threw "antibiotics" in there. Antibiotics were not available to the general public until after World War 2 when the death rates from infectious diseases had dramatically declined and, most significantly, antibiotics have no effect on viral diseases.*

Then comes the "but" in the Health Canada propaganda sheet: "But consider this: In 1981, Sweden cut immunization for whooping cough (pertussis) because of fears about the vaccine. In about four years, the annual rate of pertussis per 100,000 children under age 6 increased from 700 cases to 3,200."

Sweden has always struck me as being a particularly enlightened country. No doubt they had good reason to stop the pertussis vaccine as we will see when we look at 'side-effects'. But the statement about increased rate interests me. *Note they don't talk about the death rate but about the number of cases. Using <u>morbidity</u> figures rather than <u>mortality</u> figures is a giant red herring and one to be aware of when reading reports from health authorities. They also ignore the cyclical nature of epidemics of infectious disease.* For example, whooping cough outbreaks tend to occur every 3-4 years; you can make figures seem to rise by quoting statistics in say, year one and year four during an outbreak and thus make it look as though there has been a sudden increase in incidence.

---

[80] *Health! Canada Magazine*, March 2001

Hilary Butler[81] quotes from a 1989 article in *International Journal of Health Services* by McKinlay, McKinlay and Beaglehole who reviewed the evidence concerning the impact of medical measures on mortality and morbidity in the United States in the 1900s. "Clearly, the medical measures considered for tuberculosis, typhoid, measles and scarlet fever were introduced at the point when the death rate for each of these diseases was already negligible. Any changes in the rates of decline that occurred subsequent to the interventions could only be minute. Of the remaining five diseases (excluding smallpox with its negligible contribution), poliomyelitis is the only disease for which the medical measures produced any noticeable change in the trends. The other four diseases – pneumonia, influenza, whooping cough, and diphtheria – exhibit relatively smooth mortality trends that are unaffected by the medical measures, even though these measures were introduced when the death rates were still notable."

[Note to self: locate the article and send multiple copies to Health Canada.]

Chickenpox

Chickenpox is defined in my 1972 *Encyclopedia and Dictionary of Medicine and Nursing* as "an acute communicable disease of childhood caused by a virus with mild constitutional symptoms and a maculopapular vesicular skin eruption; also called varicella. It is a common childhood disease and is rarely severe. One attack usually gives immunity."

Children with chickenpox suffer with a slight fever, headache, backache and loss of appetite for a day or two before small, red spots appear, usually on the back or chest. These spots enlarge and turn into vesicles filled with clear fluid. After a day or two, scabs form and these peel off in anything from five to 20 days. Treatment is bed rest, lots of water and calamine lotion to relieve itching of the spots.

In the US, there are about 50 deaths a year from chickenpox in adults and children. Out of 400 million people this is a low risk; a person has a greater chance of being struck by lightning in the US as 90 people a year die from that cause. Nevertheless the FDA approved a varicella vaccine in March, 1995.

The same virus that is said to cause chickenpox, *varicella-zoster virus* (VZV), is also said to cause herpes zoster (shingles). A person who has never had chicken pox cannot get shingles. After a bout of chicken pox, the VZV lies dormant in the body's cranial nerve and dorsal root ganglia and if VZV immunity declines below a certain threshold, shingles breaks out. Repeated exposure to chickenpox in the community ensures the maintenance of VZV immunity.[82]

Shingles may cause excruciating pain, so bad that it can be mistaken for kidney stones or a heart attack depending on which nerves are involved. Shingles can cause hearing loss, blindness, facial paralysis, bladder impairment and long-

---

[81] Butler H & P, *Just a Little Prick.* Robert Reisinger Memorial Trust, New Zealand, 2006

[82] Givner, C. & Goldman, GS. *Injection.* Medical Veritas International Inc. 2006

term, debilitating pain. Based on five years of data the Centers for Disease Control (CDC) estimated that 75% of medical costs due to VZV was spent on shingles.

Gary Goldman, Ph.D, Research Analyst with the CDC, followed the chickenpox figures after the introduction of the vaccine in 1995. For five years he reported positive and welcome results. But in 2000 he discovered serious side-effects. This time his reports were not welcome and he was told to "cease and desist from publishing in a medical journal."[83] He resigned from the Varicella Active Surveillance Project in 2002.

Goldman told the CDC that adult exposure to childhood chickenpox provided an immunological boost to help postpone or protect against shingles. If childhood chickenpox were to be eradicated this natural protection against shingles would be lost. His warning went unheeded until chickenpox broke out in a vaccinated elementary school. This event prompted the CDC to order a retrospective study conducted by Yih et al. They found a 90% increase in the incidence of shingles in the adult population of Massachusetts.[84]

Fear not, for there is now a vaccine for shingles. Approved in 2006, Zostavax, according to the package insert, contains MSG, gelatine, neomycin and bovine calf serum as well as aborted fetal tissue (MRC-5 cells) among other things.[85] The MRC-5 cell line was derived from normal lung tissue of a 14-week old aborted fetus.[86] In other words, although the lung tissue might have been normal, the cells came from dead human flesh.

A Johns Hopkins Medicine article on prescription drugs informs us that "The vaccine has not been studied in people who have had shingles, and little is known about whether it works in people younger than sixty. It is not clear how long immunity lasts. People with a weakened immune system caused by treatments like radiation or corticosteroids or who have leukemia, lymphoma, or untreated tuberculosis should not get the vaccine."

I have not had shingles and I am over 60 but there is no way I will allow anyone to inject dead human tissue and serum from a calf, with all its DNA and whatever else, into my bloodstream.

Why was a vaccine necessary for a harmless childhood disease? Who decides that a disease is a public health hazard requiring preventive measures? It used to be Public Health professionals; now it appears to be the pharmaceutical industry. Is a shingles epidemic in adults too high a price to pay for attempting to prevent children from getting a mild childhood disease? When thousands of adults become sick, will the varicella vaccine be held responsible or will the epidemic of shingles simply be "coincidental"?

---

[83] Ibid.
[84] Morbidly and Mortality Weekly Reports. May 2004
[85] www.merck.com
[86] www.olympusfluoview.com

Tetanus

Tetanus is not a childhood disease, nor is it contagious. Nevertheless, a vaccine for it is given routinely to children combined with the ones for diphtheria and pertussis (whooping cough.) Is it coincidental that these three diseases are caused by the toxins produced in association with germs, not the germs themselves?

Tetanus, also known as lockjaw, is caused by an anaerobic bacillus, *clostridium tetani.* The bacilli are found on the surface of the body, in the mouth, in household dust, clothing, and particularly in cultivated soil. Normally harmless, they will thrive where there is dirt and no oxygen such as in deep puncture wounds. In these anaerobic conditions the bacilli flourish and the body produces toxins that affect the nervous system. We have all heard of the dangers of stepping on a rusty nail. Tetanus develops when drainage of a wound is blocked and dirt remains in the tissues. The obvious prevention is to make sure deep wounds drain and are clean.

Unlike infectious diseases, people who have had tetanus are *not immune* to it. If natural immunity cannot be acquired, how can artificial immunity from a vaccine?

The diphtheria and tetanus vaccine administered to infants and children contain thimerosal (mercury) and aluminium phosphate, both known to be neurotoxins.

In the US, deaths from tetanus numbered 28,065 in 1901, 4709 in 1931 and 1697 in 1946 when the vaccine was introduced. In England the death rate from tetanus is shown in the following graph:

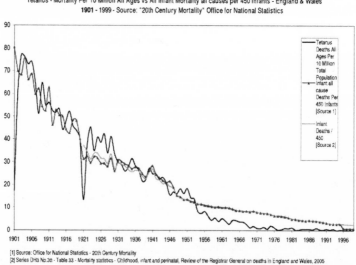

Tetanus - Mortality Per 10 Million All Ages vs All Infant Mortality all causes per 450 infants - England & Wales
1901 - 1999 - Source: "20th Century Mortality" Office for National Statistics

[1] Source: Office for National Statistics - 20th Century Mortality
[2] Series DH3 No.38 - Table 33 - Mortality statistics - Childhood, infant and perinatal, Review of the Registrar General on deaths in England and Wales, 2005
070725

The graphs shown above make it perfectly clear that vaccines had nothing to do with the falling death rates from childhood disease. Yet many people believe that if there were no vaccines we would succumb to "deadly", catastrophic outbreaks of measles or chicken pox or mumps.

"But what about polio?" my friends ask. So what about polio?

Polio

I was a student nurse in the fifties during a polio epidemic. I don't remember seeing any cases of polio in our hospital but I do remember two 'iron lungs' gathering dust in the corridor leading to the chapel. They resembled giant, metal coffins on wheeled legs and where the head would be, a platform extended to support a pillow. I don't think they were ever used in my time as by then Boyle's respirators had been invented. These two-tiered carts holding small tanks of oxygen, air and nitrous oxide, regulated by glass flow meters, artificially controlled respiration through a tube in the mouth.

In 1887 Sweden experienced an epidemic of paralytic polio and the first large epidemic in the US began in 1893 in Boston. The disease became a major problem in 1907-1916 , with an outbreak that affected 26 states.[87]

In the 1920s, disproportionate attention was paid to polio in the United States because Franklin Roosevelt suffered from the paralytic form of the disease. His wealth and status allowed him to form the Georgia Warm Springs Foundation for the treatment of polio.[88] This foundation won large, tax-free grants to experiment with treatments and conduct research. In 1938, Roosevelt announced the formation of a non-partisan group to be called the National Foundation for Infantile Paralysis. From this sprang the March of Dimes, which asked every citizen to send a dime directly to the president to support the Foundation.

I mention these snippets of history because polio always comes up in a discussion about vaccines as though polio was a disease that ravaged the North American continent. In actual fact, the number of deaths in the US in 1936 from polio was 3666, compared to 6809 from whooping cough and 8449 from influenza.[89]

Unlike other infectious diseases that are usually correlated with poverty, poor sanitation and malnutrition, polio occurred with the greatest frequency in countries with advanced hygiene. To explain this apparent paradox, an American physician and nutritionist, Dr. Benjamin Sandler, offered the theory that polio is related to low blood sugar in the human body caused, funnily enough, by eating too much sweet and starchy food. During an epidemic in North Carolina in 1948, Dr. Sandler campaigned to have people follow a sugarless, low carbohydrate diet. As a result North Carolina experienced the greatest reduction in the number of cases in the whole country: their case rate of 66.3 in 1948 fell to 6.3 in 1949.[90] North

---

[87] Vermeulen, F. *Monera*. Emryss Publishers, 2005, p.678

[88] Oshinsky, DM. *Polio: An American Story*. Oxford University Press, 2005

[89] Alderson, M. *International Mortality Statistics*, 1981

[90] Diet is a Major Factor in Polio Prevention, Dr. Sandler Believes. *The Asheville Citizen*, August 5, 1948

Carolina's example was not followed largely because of the outcries from soft drink and ice-cream manufacturers.

Polio deaths in the US were 7229 in 1921, and down to 3539 in 1941. In 1956, when deaths from polio were down to 1604, the vaccine was introduced. In the UK, an epidemic of polio peaked in 1950 and had declined by 82% by 1956, at which time the vaccine was introduced.[91] After that the rate of decline remained virtually the same.

Three types of polio vaccine have been used: the first, developed by Salk, consisted of 'killed' polio viruses and was administered by injection; the second, developed by Sabin, was made of 'live' polio viruses and administered orally; the third, eIPV, consisted of 'killed' polio viruses that had been cultured in human cells rather than in monkey kidneys.[92] (Yet virology textbooks tell us that viruses are inert and not alive.)

The first large scale trial of the Salk polio vaccine started in the US on April 26, 1954 when 440,000 children were vaccinated. A year later the American public rejoiced at the manufacture of a safe and efficient vaccine and Salk became a national hero. And, of course, Hollywood wanted to make a movie about his life.

The joy was short-lived. Dr. M. B. Bayly, M.R.C.S., L.R.C.P. wrote in 1956:[93] "Only thirteen days after the vaccine had been acclaimed by the whole of the American press and radio, as one of the greatest medical discoveries of the century, and after the English Minister of Health had announced he would go ahead with the manufacture of the vaccine, came the first news of disaster. Children inoculated with one brand of vaccine had developed poliomyelitis. In the following days more and more cases were reported, some of them after inoculation with other brands of the vaccine. Then came another, and wholly unlooked for complication. The Denver Medical Officer, Dr. Florio, announced the development of what he called "satellite" polio, that is, cases of the disease in the parents or other close contacts of the children who had been inoculated and, after a few days' illness in hospital, had returned home; they communicated the disease to others, although not suffering from it themselves."

How history repeats itself. Weren't there similar stories about the inoculation of smallpox pus in the 18th century? An article in *Time* (May 30, 1955) commented: "In retrospect, a good deal of the blame for the vaccine fiasco also went to the National Foundation, which, with years of publicity had built up the danger of polio out of all proportion to its actual incidence and had rushed into vaccinations this year with patently insufficient preparation."

According to Dr. Dennis Geffern, OBE, MD, DPH, "of every 100 people who become infected with the (polio) virus, 90% remain symptomless; 9% show some slight sign of the disease such as sore throat or stiffness of the neck, whilst

---

[91] Obomsawin, R. Immunization: a Report for CIDA, May ,1992
[92] Null, G. *Vaccines: a Second Opinion*. www.garynull.com
[93] Bayly, MB. The Story of the Salk Anti-Poliomyelitis Vaccine. whale.to/vaccine/bayly.html

only 1% develop definite paralysis."[94] He is reported in *Public Health* (March 1955) to have told the Metropolitan Branch of the Society of Medical Officers of Health, that "we are apt to forget that poliomyelitis is the least serious of all infectious diseases with the exception of that one complication, or extension of the disease, which destroys motor cells in the brain and spinal cord and causes paralysis. Apart from this it appears to be a mild infection lasting a few days, the symptoms of which are probably less serious than a cold in the head and from which recovery is complete and immunity, lasting. If we could be sure that an individual contracting poliomyelitis would not become paralysed then there might be much to be said for spreading the disease in order that a community might develop natural immunity."

Persevering with vaccines for a now man-made polio epidemic, Sabin came to the rescue with a live virus vaccine that could be administered orally. I worked in San Francisco at the time and I remember lining up with other nurses, unquestioningly, for our sugar cube. At that time, the idea that a vaccine could be harmful never occurred to us.

As is its wont, the US introduced compulsory vaccination. In 1958, the mass vaccination campaigns triggered a huge increase in the numbers of polio cases in the US and Canada. The highest increase was 700% in Ottawa. Sinclair[95] quotes figures from four States:

States	1958 Before compulsory shots	1959 After compulsory shots
North Carolina	78 cases	313 cases
Connecticut	45 cases	123 cases
Tennessee	119 cases	386 cases
Ohio	17 cases	52 cases

According to Jonas Salk, the maker of the original vaccine, the live polio vaccine developed by Sabin was "the principal, if not the sole, cause of the 140 polio cases reported in the US since 1961. At the present time the risk of acquiring polio from the live virus vaccine is greater than from naturally occurring viruses."[96]

The touching faith in the efficacy of vaccines is illustrated by the explanation for these figures from the *Los Angeles County Health Index: Morbidity and Mortality, Reportable Diseases*.

---

[94] Chaitow, L. *Vaccination and Immunization: Dangers, Delusions and Alternatives.* Saffron Walden, England, 1988

[95] Sinclair, Ian. *Vaccination: The "Hidden" Facts. Australia*, 1994

[96] Golden, I. *Vaccination? A Review of Risks and Alternatives.* Australia, 1994

DATE	VIRAL OR ASEPTIC MENINGITIS	POLIO
July 1955	50	273
July 1961	161	65
July 1963	151	31
September 1966	256	31
October 1966	312	3

The explanation for this strange inversion of figures was: "Most cases reported prior to July 1, 1958 as non-paralytic poliomyelitis are now reported as viral or aseptic meningitis," because since the vaccine had "wiped out polio", children with similar symptoms must have something else – meningitis.[97] It's the re-naming game again.

Burton reported at an international health convention in 1978 that data compiled by the University of New South Wales revealed that polio immunization programs had no measurable impact in reversing what was a recent epidemic. He explained that polio comes in cycles anyway and when it does subside, it is inadvertently considered "conquered" by vaccines.[98]

Dr. Bernard Greenberg, (former Dean, School of Public Health, University of North Carolina) testified at the Congressional Hearings on polio vaccines in 1962.[99] He said, "As a result of ... changes in both diagnosis and diagnostic methods, the rates of paralytic poliomyelitis plummeted from the early 1950s to a low in 1957."

These changes were:
• Redefinition of what constitutes an epidemic
• Redefinition of the disease
• Mislabelling, and later reclassification (before 1954 "large numbers" of presumed "paralytic polio" cases became "Coxsakie and aseptic meningitis cases.")

A medical panel moderated at the 120th Annual Meeting of the Illinois State Medical Society confirmed that in 1959 roughly 1,000 cases of paralytic polio occurred in persons who had previously received multiple doses of the Salk vaccine. As a panel member, Dr. Greenberg said, "One of the most obvious pieces of misinformation is the 50% rise in paralytic poliomyelitis in 1958, and the real accelerated increase in 1959, have been caused by persons failing to be vaccinated. This represents an unwillingness to face facts and to evaluate the true effectiveness of the Salk vaccine."

The polio vaccine may not have been successful but the publicity campaign certainly was; people still believe that there was a dangerous epidemic of polio in the fifties and that the disease was eliminated by a vaccine.

---

[97] Kent, C. The Polio Vaccine Myth. *The Chiropractic Journal,* March 2000
[98] Obomsawin, R. Immunization: a Report for CIDA, May ,1992
[99] Obomsawin, R. Universal Immunization: Medical Miracle or Masterful Mirage? www.whale/to

The last word on polio vaccination belongs to Mendelsohn.

"There is an ongoing debate amongst the immunologists regarding the killed virus vs. live virus vaccine. Supporters of the killed virus vaccine maintain that it is the presence of live virus organisms in the other product that is responsible for the polio cases that appear. Supporters of the live virus type argue that the killed virus vaccine offers inadequate protection and actually increases the susceptibility (to polio) of those vaccinated. This affords me a rare opportunity to be comfortably neutral. I believe that both factions are right and that use of either of the vaccines will increase, not diminish, the possibility that your child will contract the disease. In short, it appears that the most effective way to protect your child from polio is to make sure that he doesn't get the vaccine."[100]

---

[100] Mendelsohn, RS. *How to raise a healthy child in spite of your doctor.* Random House, 1984

Chapter 8

The Side Effects of DPT

Lycosa tarantula, a wolf spider, is found in Italy and Spain. Although a vicious-looking creature, its bite does not kill but can affect the motor and sensory neuro-systems. A bitten person exhibits a bizarre restlessness that gave rise to the dance aptly called the tarantella. In addition to uncontrolled agitation, the bite causes excessive sensitivity to light and colour, and aggravation by noise, facial pallor, and enlarged glands.

As a person in charge of treatment you have a patient with a bright red face. You note that spider venom causes pallor and you want to treat this patient's face. You administer tarantula extract. The face pales but your patient dances madly, has to wear sunglasses all the time, is deafened by rustling paper and has swollen glands. These then, are "side-effects".

You then treat the restlessness with a drug recommended by Big Pharma, called Koolit. Your patient calms down but the side-effect of Koolit is an embarrassing pubic rash that he can't stop scratching. So you give Dermacease. That stops the rash but the side-effect of Dermacease is … And so it goes on. This is the mindset that governs the practice of modern medicine and is one I didn't grow up with.

The damage done by vaccines is so profound that it's difficult to know where to begin. Although each can cause damage, perhaps the worst is the pertussis vaccine.

Two of the first people to raise the alarm, Coulter and Fisher, wrote in *A Shot in the Dark*, "One of the strangest elements in the pertussis vaccine story is that the vaccine was introduced on a mass scale in England, the United States and other industrialized countries of the world without a systematic effort to evaluate its side effects. Once vaccination programs were in full swing in developed countries, almost no attempt was made to adequately monitor side effects or improve the safety of the vaccine."[101]

---

[101] Coulter, HL & Fisher, BL. *A Shot in the Dark.* Avery Publishing Group Inc. 1991

From 1942-1944, controlled trials were conducted in Oxford. The results of these trials? Vaccines were ineffective because no significant difference was observed in the incidence or severity of whooping cough between the vaccinated and unvaccinated children.[102]

In 1947 the British Medical Council began testing the pertussis vaccine on 50,000 children despite the results of the previous trials and despite the fact that the incidence of whooping cough was rapidly declining. All the children in the test were 14 months old or older; not newborns. Eight children had convulsions within 72 hours of the shot; 34 within 28 days of the shot. The doctors denied a possible connection saying that there was no reason to consider that the convulsions were precipitated by the vaccine.[103]

In 1948 Byers and Moll of the Harvard medical school examined 15 children who had reacted violently within 72 hours of a pertussis vaccination. All the children had been normal prior to the shot. None had had a convulsion before. Of the 15, two died and nine suffered neurological damage. One child became blind, deaf, spastic and helpless.[104]

Once again the data were ignored and vaccination programs continued. I sometimes wonder whether if you slapped these people across the face with a wet kipper, they would deny the presence of fish. The United States then started vaccinating newborns even though the preliminary trial was conducted on children no younger than 14 months and despite the convulsions.

Sweden was naughty. In 1960 Ström, writing in the *British Medical Journal*, stated, "In Sweden the incidence of neurological complications after pertussis does not appear to be as high as that after vaccination."[105] He also pointed out that whooping cough had become a much milder disease and questioned whether universal vaccination is justified. This is the country that Health Canada chastises in its propaganda. No child has died of pertussis in Sweden since 1970, notwithstanding the cessation of DPT vaccine.

There is a wide range of estimates about the frequency of damage caused by the DPT (diphtheria, pertussis, tetanus) vaccine. On one hand the British Department of Health and Social Security reckon that only 1 in 300,000 vaccinates exhibit permanent neurological damage.[106] Other researchers estimate that permanent damage occurs in 1 in 300. Between these two extremes, Cornoyer's[107]

---

[102] Scheibner, V. *Vaccination: 100 Years of Orthodox Research Shows that Vaccination Represents a Medical Assault on the Immune System.* New Atlantean Press, 1993 p.14

[103] Ibid.

[104] Byers, RK & Moll, FC. Encephalopathies following prophylactic pertussis vaccination. *Paediatrics.* 1(4):437-56

[105] Ström, J. Is universal vaccination against pertussis always justified? *British Medical Journal,* October 22, 1960

[106] Obomaswin R. Immunization: a Report for CIDA, May ,1992

[107] Cornoyer, C. *What About Immunizations? A Parents Guide to Informed Decision-making.* Private Research Publication, Canby, Oregon, 1987

research findings in *A Parent's Guide to Vaccination*, suggest the following reactions:

Persistent crying – 1 in 20
High fever – 1 in 66
High-pitched screaming – 1 in 180
Convulsions – 1 in 350
Shock-like condition or collapse – 1 in 22,000
Permanent brain damage – 1 in 62,000
Death – 1 in 71,600

If parents were properly informed of these risks would they line up their children for their 'shots' so readily? The statistics, hundreds of them, are there for the reading but to me, they don't mean as much as a personal story. And there are plenty of those to choose from. One of the most poignant, "*Death by Lethal Vaccine Injection*" by Christine Colebeck can be read on the web.

Stories like this are dismissed as "anecdotal", in contrast to the "scientific data" health authorities reputedly use. The word used to disconnect a convulsion from the administration of a vaccine is "coincidental," i.e. the convulsion would have occurred anyway. No one has studied this, of course. And who would fund such a study?

Christine Colebeck was told that her baby died of Sudden Infant Death Syndrome – SIDS. One of every 500 US births ends in a death from SIDS according to the FDA's own statistics. That translates into 7000 babies a year.

I turn to Dr. Viera Scheibner, an Australian, who has written two influential books: *Vaccination: 100 Years of Orthodox Research Shows that Vaccines Represent a Medical Assault on the Immune System*, and *Behavioural Problems in Childhood: the Link to Vaccination*. As I come from a culture that calls a spade a spade – that is, from Yorkshire – I like Viera because she does not mince words. I envision visiting her in her home office, a book-lined room with sun streaming through the window. I have seen her photograph. She is about my age, perhaps slightly younger, with hazel eyes set in a wisdom-lined face and similar 'pudgy' hands to mine. The dialogue I have ascribed to her is taken from her books and used with her permission.

*   *   *

JC. I was so sorry to miss your visit to our area in 2000. I had just had a hip replacement and was still immobile. Can you tell me how you became interested in vaccination?

VS. Yes. On October 12, 1985 my life changed profoundly. On that day I met Leif Karlsson, a biomedical electronics engineer specialising in patient monitoring systems. I asked him to develop a breathing monitor for babies.

JC. Who would use such a monitor?

VS. Mostly Cotwatch went to parents wishing to monitor their newborn baby's breathing.

JC. Cotwatch? In North America that would be Cribwatch, I guess.

VS. We decided to rent the first 150 units and to keep in close contact with the parents who used them. Soon, some twenty units were out there working and some time later parents starting ringing us to report that Cotwatch was sounding alarms. Clusters of five to seven short alarms sounded within about a 15 minute period.

JC. What would trigger the alarm?

VS. They occurred after the baby had been exposed to stress, or happened a day or two before the child went down with a common cold or cut its first tooth.

JC. Did the alarm mean the baby had stopped breathing?

VS. Most of them indicated that they were breathing very shallowly. In most cases no intervention was needed as the babies spontaneously resumed normal (deeper) breathing. Others were 'near-miss' babies, babies who stopped breathing, were found in time and successfully resuscitated.

JC. The monitor must be a boon to anxious parents. It also sounds like a wonderful research opportunity.

VS. We couldn't find a paediatrician who would undertake independent research to elucidate and further develop ideas based on initial observations with Cotwatch, so we decided to do the necessary data collection and research ourselves.

Without endeavouring to do so specifically, we recorded the breathing of babies before and after they were vaccinated. The pattern of breathing that emerged over the days and weeks was highly significant. It showed that babies' breathing was affected in a certain characteristic manner over a long period of time following DPT injection.

JC. You didn't realise that vaccination is a hotly debated topic?

VS. No. We saw only that DPT vaccination caused babies a lot of stress and sometimes major flare-ups over a period of at least 45-60 days following injections. When we showed the records to paediatricians they pointed to the arrow indicating day zero (when the DPT injection was administered) and commented without hesitation: "This is the cause."

JC. And they still weren't interested in doing the research?

VS. No, we were forced to start our own search for the truth. Several years later I had collected just about every most quoted publication written on the subject of the effectiveness and dangers of vaccines, and more. Supported by data from our continuing research with the Cotwatch breathing monitor, I decided to write a concise and brief summary of my literature search, reviewing many thousands of pages of scientific journals and other publications I had studied.

JC. I have talked about vaccine damage in my book. I am particularly interested in the connection between DPT and SIDS. Your book presents several pages of review of studies of infants who have died within days of a DPT shot. Yet the conclusions drawn from these studies seem to vary a great deal. Physicians acknowledged a time, a temporal relationship, but not a causal one.

*VS. Speaking of a **temporal** relationship between DPT injections and cot death, as opposed to a **causal** relationship, is totally inappropriate semantics. It would be just too much of a coincidence that tens of thousands of babies die after DPT injections, yet none of these deaths would be caused by such a highly noxious substance as DPT vaccine. This is especially instructive since the vast majority of these babies were healthy bouncing infants just hours before they were injected with DPT and died.*

JC. What did your Cotwatch computer printouts show?

VS. Non-stop monitoring during sleep showed a marked change in the pattern and duration of events in breathing after the injection.

JC. Is there any doubt that there's a causal relationship between DPT vaccination and SIDS?

VS. The question has, quite adequately and indeed without a shadow of a doubt, been resolved by the Japanese experience with cot death.

JC. What was that?

VS. When they moved the vaccination age to two years, the entity of cot death disappeared and the overall infant mortality rate fell markedly. Japan zoomed from 17th (very high mortality rate) to first place in the world, (lowest mortality rate).

JC. Thank you, Dr. Scheibner. One last question: after your extensive review of the conventional medical journals like The Lancet, what is your conclusion?

VS. There is no evidence whatsoever that vaccines of any kind – but especially those against childhood diseases – are effective in preventing the infectious diseases they are supposed to prevent. Further, adverse effects are amply documented and are far more significant to public health than any adverse effects of infectious diseases.

*   *   *   **

In the USA, the cost of a single DPT shot rose from 11 cents in 1982 to $11.40 in 1987. This 1000% increase was to allow $8 per shot to cover legal costs incurred by parents of brain-damaged children or of children who died after vaccination.[108]

As if it is not tragic enough that 7000 babies are found dead in their cribs every year in the US, parents, particularly fathers, are at risk of being accused of shaking their baby to death. At present there is an "epidemic" of so-called "shaken baby syndrome", a condition that is causing great concern in social workers and public health nurses who are blind to the connection between dead babies and vaccination.

While incidents of child abuse undoubtedly occur, why is there such a huge increase in the numbers of adults with a desire to batter their babies? What else can cause brain swelling, intracranial bleeding, retinal haemorrhages and fractured skulls? Since mass vaccination of infants began the medical literature is full of reports of brain disorders.

Vaccines, like the pertussis vaccine, are actually used to induce encephalomyelitis in experimental animals. This condition is characterized by brain swelling and haemorrhaging to the same extent found in "shaken" babies. As Scheibner says, "When lab animals develop symptoms of vaccine damage and then die, it is never considered coincidental; but when children develop the same symptoms and die after the administration of the same vaccines, it *is* considered

---

[108] Sinclair, Ian. *Vaccination: The "Hidden" Facts.* Australia, 1992

coincidental or caused by their parents or other care givers. When all this fails, then it is considered *mysterious*."[109]

An eighteen-month old child recently died in my community. I was told that his immune system had collapsed but the doctors didn't know why. When I asked if he had been vaccinated, my question was greeted with astonishment. The idea that vaccines can cause harm is so foreign that the idea simply does not enter a person's head. I don't know the answer to my question but I am willing to bet that the child's problems could be tied to the vaccinations he was given and progressed from there. Nevertheless, that connection would be, of course, dismissed as coincidental.

---

[109] Scheibner, V. Shaken Baby Syndrome – the vaccination link. *Nexus Magazine*, Aug/Sept, 1998

Chapter 9

Further Vaccine Side Effects

"You should learn not to make personal remarks," Alice said with some severity. "It's very rude."

The Hatter opened his eyes very wide on hearing this; but all he said was, "Why is a raven like a writing desk?"

Come, we shall have some fun now, thought Alice. I'm glad they've begun asking riddles. "I believe I can answer that," she added aloud.

Dr. Rieu offered a solution. "Because there's a 'B' in 'Both'?"[110]

The Mad Hatter was not merely a whimsical character of Carrols; when *Alice in Wonderland* was published in 1865, the expression 'mad as a hatter' was commonplace. The term arose from an occupational disease.

Top hats, made of felt, were once very popular in both North America and Europe. The best were made from beaver fur, the cheapest from rabbit. Cheaper furs were first brushed with a solution of mercury compound to roughen the fibres and make them mat more easily, a process called 'carroting' because it made the fur turn orange. (Beaver fur had natural serrated edges so this step was unnecessary.) As hatters worked in poorly ventilated workshops, when they used rabbit they breathed in the mercury and accumulated it in their bodies.[111]

Mercury is a cumulative neurotoxin that affects 6 body systems: gut, brain, eyes, muscle control, immune system and speech. At one time common household remedies like mercurochrome and teething powder also caused acute mercury poisoning. These products are now off the market. Currently, the major sources or mercury are seafood, environmental pollution and dental amalgams. If we ingest mercury, the body has a survival mechanism in the form of bile. Although bile's main job is to prepare fats for digestion, it also soaks up mercury and transports it out through the digestive system. Bile, however, is not formed until 6 years of age and therefore children cannot expel mercury, so it accumulates in them.

Here are some facts about mercury:[112]

---

[110] Carrol, Lewis. The Annotated Alice with notes by Martin Gardner. Bramhall House, 1960

[111] Quinion, M. www.worldwidewords.org

[112] http://pediatrics.aappublications.org

0.5 parts per billion (ppb) mercury = kills human neuroblastoma cells.[113]
2 ppb mercury = US Environmental Protection Agency (EPA) limit for drinking water.[114]
20 ppb mercury = neurite membrane structure destroyed.[115]
200 ppb mercury = level in liquid the EPA classifies as hazardous waste.[116]

And then you have the vaccines.

25,000 ppb mercury = concentration of mercury in the Hepatitis B vaccine, administered at birth in the US from 1990 – 2001.
50,000 ppb mercury = concentration of mercury in multi-dose DTaP and Haemophilus B vaccine vials, administered 4 times each in the 1990's to children at 2, 4, 6, 12 and 18 months of age.
50,000 ppb mercury is the current "preservative" level of mercury in multi-dose flu, meningococcal and tetanus vaccines (given to 7years and older). This can be confirmed by simply checking the information given by the manufacturers with the multi-dose vials.

The safe levels of mercury, set by the US Environmental Protection Agency (EPA), are 0.1 mcg/kg/day. Through vaccinations American children receive 237 micrograms. On the day of birth they are given 12 mcg of mercury in a hepatitis B shot. In 1997 hepatitis B cases numbered 10,000 in the US with 306 cases occurring in children under fourteen. The only babies at risk of Hepatitis B are those born to women with it, but the vaccine is given routinely to all babies.

In 1996, out of 3.9 millions births, 54 cases of hepatitis B in the 0 to 1 age group were reported to the Centers for Disease Control, making an observed incidence of 0.001 percent. In 1996 alone, 1,080 adverse reactions to the vaccine occurred in the 0 to 1 age group including 47 deaths.[117] So in one year there were 54 cases of hepatitis B in infants, 54 cases that the authorities reckon a vaccine is needed to prevent and, in the same year, there were 47 deaths and another 1,033 adverse reactions from the vaccine.

Thimerosal—a form of mercury used as a preservative in vaccines—has powerful toxic effects for several reasons: first, it is injected straight into the bloodstream; there is no blood-brain barrier in infants and, as mentioned earlier, infants don't produce bile and organic mercury like thimerosal converts *irreversibly* into its inorganic form when it reaches nerve tissue.[118] Furthermore,

---

[113] Parran et al., *Toxicol Sci* 2005; 86: 132-140
[114] http://www.epa.gov/safewater/contaminants/index.html11#mcls
[115] Leong et al., *Neurorreport* 2002: 12:733-37
[116] http://www.epa.gov/epaoswer/hazwaste/mercury/regs.htm#hazwaste
[117] Givner, C & Goldman, GS. *Injection*. Medical Veritas International Inc. 2006
[118] Bernard, S. et al. Autism: a novel form of mercury poisoning. www.mercola.com

the myelin sheath that protects nerves is not formed until two years of age, meaning in younger children the infant's nerves are exposed.

There is now increasing suspicion that thimerosal causes autism. Autism was first described in 1943 in children born in the 1930s. Thimerosal was introduced into vaccines in the 1930s. Prior to 1970, autism prevalence was 1:2000. From 1970 – 1990 (during a period of increased use of vaccines containing thimerosal) the ratio rose to 1:1000. In the late 1980s and early 1990s, two more mercury-laced vaccines, the HiB and Hepatitis B, were added to the recommended vaccination schedule for children. The autism rate in the US in 2006 was 1:166 according to the Centers for Disease Control.

One researcher, Sallie Bernard and her group, compared the signs and symptoms of mercury poisoning with those of autism and showed that every major characteristic of autism was exhibited in cases of documented mercury poisoning. [119] When the signs and symptoms of one condition are the same as another it is reasonable to think there is a connection.

In 1992 the FDA ordered that thimerosal be taken out of dog vaccines. [120]

In 1998 the FDA stated that "over-the-counter drug products containing thimerosal and other mercury forms are not generally recognized as safe and effective." [121]

Then contradictorily in 2000, the FDA pronounced that "vaccines have safe levels of mercury." [122]

Senator Robert F. Kennedy, JR. wrote a fascinating exposé of a government cover-up of a study announced at a CDC convened meeting in June 2000. The study showed a definite link between thimerosal and autism. According to CDC epidemiologist, Tom Verstraeten, who had analysed the agency's database of 100,000 children, thimerosal appeared to be responsible for a dramatic increase in autism and other neurological disorders such as speech delays, hyperactivity and attention-deficit disorder. Since 1991, when the CDC and the FDA recommended three more vaccines laced with thimerosal for very young infants – one given within hours of birth – the number of cases of autism increased fifteenfold, from 1:2500 to 1:166. [123]

Instead of alerting the public or ensuring withdrawal of the vaccines, officials and executives at this meeting spent two days discussing how to cover up the damaging data. The CDC paid the Institute of Medicine to conduct a new study to rule out the metal's link to autism. And in order to thwart the Freedom of

---

[119] Ibid.

[120] O'Shea, T. *The Sanctity of Human Blood: Vaccination I$ not Immunization.* Two Trees, San Jose, California, 2004

[121] Ibid.

[122] O'Shea, T. Autism and mercury: the San Diego Conference. www.thedoctorwithin.com

[123] Kennedy, RF. Deadly Immunity. *Rolling Stone*, June 20, 2005. www.whale.to/vaccine/kennedy.html

Information Act, it gave its database to a private company so that it was unavailable to independent researchers.

So that the *vaccine manufacturers would not suffer a financial loss*, the CDC and FDA made available the dangerous vaccines for export to developing countries. And so that the *vaccine manufacturers would not suffer legally*, Senator Bill Frist – a recipient of $873,000 from the pharmaceutical industry – worked to create laws under the Homeland Security Bill that would protect vaccine makers from liability for any damage caused by their vaccines to babies!

Dr. Russell Blaylock managed to pry loose the report of the "Scientific Review of Vaccine Safety Datalink Information" as the 2000 conference was called, by invoking the Freedom of Information Act.[124] The conference was attended by 51 scientists and physicians of whom five represented vaccine manufacturers. To give some idea of how these people think, I will quote some extracts from the report.

Dr. Bernier, Associate Director for Science in the National Immunization Program of the CDC, related some pertinent history arising from an earlier meeting in 1999. He said (page 12), "In the United States, there was a growing recognition that cumulative exposure (to mercury) may exceed some of the guidelines." He is referring to three guidelines set by several regulatory agencies. He also explained that he is referring to children exposed to thimerosal in vaccines.

If developing countries are under the delusion the US is helping them out by sending them vaccines, note this statement by Dr. Johnson (page 17): "We agree that it would be desirable to remove mercury from US licensed vaccines, but we did not agree that this was a universal recommendation that we would make because of the issue concerning preservatives for delivering vaccines to other countries, particularly developing countries, in the absence of hard data that implied that there was, in fact, a problem."

So there you have it. It is desirable to remove mercury from vaccines for American kids but not for kids in developing countries who, because of poor nutrition, parasitic and bacterial infections, and low birth weight, are at a far greater risk of harm from mercury.

Even though this group were aware of the dangers of mercury, Dr. Robert Chen, chief of Vaccine Safety and Development at the National Immunization Program at the CDC, gives a hint as to why they refuse to act on page 169. "The issue is that it is impossible, unethical, to leave kids unimmunized, so you will never, ever resolve that issue. So then we have to refer back from that." What he is saying is that the immunization program is more important than the safety of the vaccines. If the problem of vaccine toxicity cannot be resolved then we must accept that some kids will be harmed.

Remember that this group met to discuss Dr. Verstraeten's discovery of alarming correlations between higher doses of thimerosal and problems with neurodevelopment, including ADD and autism. Dr. Rapin expressed her concern over what would be said when this information eventually gets out to the public.

---

[124] Blaylock, RL. The Truth Behind the Vaccine Coverup. http://articles.mercola.com

She says on page 197 that they better make sure that "a) We counsel them carefully and b) that we pursue this because of the very important public health and public implications of the data."

But, to try to prevent this information becoming public, stamped in bold letters on top of each page of Dr. Verstraeten's study were the words, "DO NOT COPY OR RELEASE" and "CONFIDENTIAL." Are these the words you might expect on a publicly funded study of vaccine safety? The answer is obvious: public awareness might endanger the vaccine program and indict the government's regulatory agencies for having ignored serious dangers to the nation's children for so many years.

On page 229, Dr. Brent, a professor of paediatrics, rails about the lawsuit problem. He tells the others that he has been involved in three lawsuits related to vaccine injuries leading to birth defects and concluded, "If you want to see junk science, look at those cases ..." On the same page, Dr. Brent admits that they are in a bad position because they have no data for their defence. So just who are the junk scientists? Those with data or those without?

Over the next 10-15 pages they discuss how to control the information so that it will not get out and, if it does, how to control the damage. Dr. Clements, the WHO representative, said, "My mandate as I sit here in this group is to make sure at the end of the day that 100,000,000 are immunized with DTP, Hepatitis B and if possible Hib, this year, next year and for many years to come, and that will have to be with thimerosal-containing vaccines unless a miracle occurs and an alternative is found quickly and is tried and found to be safe." In other words, "I don't care how harmful vaccines are; they will be given now and for ever."

In the meantime thousands of parents are left to grieve over their previously healthy children, now damaged for life. And the rest of the population is left to pay.

Dr. Verstraeten published a different version of the study in the November 2003 issue of *Pediatrics*, which did not show the statistical correlation he had presented at the conference. No explanation was provided for this discrepancy.[125]

However, after 1½ years attempting to access the database, Dr. Mark Geier and David Geier compared data for a vaccine containing thimerosal with another that used an alternative preservative, and demonstrated that the rate of autism was six times higher in the group that received the thimerosal.[126]

As the federal government worked to prevent scientists from studying the thimerosal–autism connection, a reporter, Dan Olmsted, of United Press International, undertook a study himself. He looked for children who had not been exposed to vaccines and found them in the Amish of Lancaster County, Pennsylvania who refuse to vaccinate their children. Given the population of the Amish and the autism rate in the US, Olmsted figured there should be 130 autistics among the group. He found only four. One had been exposed to mercury from a power plant; the other three had received vaccines.

[125] Kirby, D. *Evidence of Harm*. St. Martin's Press, New York, 2005, p.363

[126] Givner, C & Goldman, GS. *Injection*. Medical Veritas International Inc. 2006

A blow-by-blow account of the thimerosal/autism controversy is related by David Kirby in his 2005 book, *Evidence of Harm*. If you read it, prepare to be disturbed by the obvious corruption in government health agencies.[127] Like many others, he is only concerned with the effect of mercury and ignores other damage done by vaccines; probably because he believes that "childhood immunization was perhaps one of the greatest public health achievements of the twentieth century ..." This statement tells me that he hasn't done his homework.

An autism rate of 1:166 children prompted a Committee on Government Reform that met in 2002 to look into vaccine safety and autism. The recorded proceedings make interesting reading. For example, Congressman Dan Burton, whose grandchild is autistic, stated, "You mean to tell me since 1929 we've been using thimerosal and the only test you know of is the one that was done in 1929, and every one of those people got meningitis and died?"[128]

The outcome was not, as you might expect, a moratorium on vaccination pending further, independent studies but simply a *request* from the FDA to vaccine manufacturers asking them to stop using thimerosal. It is easy to imagine the equivalent organization in the UK talking to Big Pharma:

*   *   *

I say, chaps, would you mind awfully not using thimerosal. You see mercury is turning kids into vegetables. We hate to trouble you but please would you use something else?

When your stock piles are finished? Well, no real hurry but parents are getting a teeny bit anxious. And, you know, they may even refuse vaccinations and where would that put you?

Oh I see; you could send the stock piles to Africa? At half-price; as a goodwill gesture?

Good thinking. Well, cheery-bye. Thank you for your consideration.

*   *   *

How history repeats itself! A disastrous smallpox epidemic in Britain following mandatory vaccination in 1870-1873 led to the Crown appointing a Royal Commission on Vaccination and Smallpox. The group first met in 1889 and took seven years to listen to testimony and to compile data for its voluminous report. Hale remarks that "fourteen pounds avoirdupois of contrary evidence hurled at the heads of the pro-vaccinationist majority on the Commission failed to make a dent in their triple-plate conviction that, in spite of everything, vaccination does prevent smallpox!"[129] However, the committee did recommend that vaccination be voluntary.

Another connection between a vaccine and autism has been made; this time with the MMR (measles, mumps, rubella) vaccine. These were mild common childhood diseases in my young days, but since the advent of a vaccine health policy, the authorities have taken to classifying them as "life-threatening."

---

[127] Kirby, D. *Evidence of Harm*. St. Martin's Press, New York, 2005
[128] Ibid.
[129] Hale, A.R. *The Medical Voodoo*. Gotham House, Inc. 1935

According to the *London Sunday Herald*, several prominent British researchers say that the MMR vaccine was not adequately tested and should never have been licensed.[130] Were any vaccines adequately tested? Is injecting vaccine into mice an adequate test of something to be used in children?

Dr. Peter Fletcher, a senior medical officer at the UK Department of Health, said, "Being extremely generous, evidence on safety was very thin; being realistic there were too few patients followed-up for sufficient time. Three weeks is not enough, neither is four weeks. On the basis that effective monovalent (single dose) vaccines were available, the Committee on the Safety of Medicines could be confident that delay in granting a license would not result in a catastrophic epidemic of measles, mumps or rubella.

"Caution should have ruled the day, answers to some important questions should have been demanded and encouragement should have been given to conduct a 12-month observational study on 10-15,000 patients and a prospective monitoring program set up with a computerized primary care database. The granting of a product license was definitely premature."[131]

The MMR vaccine was banned in Japan in 1993 after 1.8 million children had been given two types of MMR and a record number developed non-viral meningitis and other adverse effects. And of the 3,969 medical compensation claims relating to vaccines in Japan in the last 30 years, 25% were made by those badly affected by the MMR vaccine.[132]

Although MMR vaccine does not contain thimerosal, Mister Andrew Wakefield – a medical doctor with the title of Mister because he's a Fellow of the Royal College of Surgeons – found the measles virus in the guts of autistic children. Autism includes not only mental disability but also severe bowel disturbances that resemble Crohn's disease. The children in the sample had not had natural measles and therefore the virus could only have come from the vaccine.

Mr. Wakefield published his results in *Lancet* in 1998. It was career suicide; MMR 'uptake' fell in the UK; *Lancet* disowned the article and Mr. Wakefield in 2007 came up before the General Medical Council (GMC) for conducting "inadequately founded" research.[133] Parents of autistic children, suspecting a link between their child's condition and the MMR vaccine, had created a fund to conduct research and hired Mr. Wakefield. Therefore, it was alleged before the GMC, Mr. Wakefield had a conflict of interest.

In March, 2009, Mr. Wakefield was still before the GMC. Although no children were hurt, the GMC was now considering charges levelled by a single complainant, Brian Deer, a journalist for *The Times* who allegedly has also been reporting this case as if he had not levelled the charges! It is one of the most basic tenets of the British, and other juridical systems, that the accused should be able to face his or her accuser and question them about their motives, vested interests and

---

[130] Day, P. *Health Wars*. Credence Publications, 2001
[131] Ibid.
[132] Ibid.
[133] BBC News, 2006/06/12

whether they have worked for or been aided in making the complaint by any other party. This has not happened. Brian Deer was not called as a witness. Andrew Wakefield now runs a clinic for autistic children in Houston, Texas. He awaits his verdict from the British Medical Council.

I remember *The Times* when it had advertisements on the front page. I grew up believing it was a high class newspaper. Now, after its malicious witch-hunt of Dr. Wakefield, I believe it has joined the worst of the gutter press. It is also extremely serious that 12 of the 36 members of the British Committee on Safety of Medicines, the equivalent of the FDA, have financial links with the MMR manufacturers.[134]

The Journal of Medical Virology in 2006 reported a government-sponsored study that concluded there is no evidence of measles virus in MMR-vaccinated autistic children. The report stated, "Contrary to the findings of some earlier studies, measles virus genetic material was not detected in the blood of MMR-vaccinated autistic children." Of course it wasn't; Mr. Wakefield found it in the gut, not the blood.

Dr. John O'Leary, a molecular biologist from Dublin, upheld Mr. Wakefield's findings. Using state-of-the-art molecular biological technologies and 'blinded protocol', where each sample was given unique numbers so that the scientists performing the investigation did not know from whom the samples came, O'Leary's team found 24 of 25 (96%) autistic children were positive for measles virus. Of the control children, who did not have autism, one of 15 (6.6%) was positive for measles virus.

On May 29, 2006, three sources [135] reported that the vaccine strain of measles virus had been found in the guts of 85% of autistic children in a New York University School of Medicine study.

The mechanism by which autism can be caused by the measles vaccine was presented by Dr. Vijendra Singh.[136] He identified specific antibodies that produce an autoimmune attack on brain tissue as a response to measles vaccine.

---

[134] Day, P. *Health Wars.* Credence Publications, 2001

[135] TimesOnline,co.uk, Telegraph.co.uk, Association of American Physicians and Surgeons.

[136] Singh, VK, Sheren, XL, Yang, VC. Serological association of measles virus and human herpesvirus-6 with brain autoantibodies in autism. *Clinical Immunology and Immunopathology*, 1998; 89(1):105-8

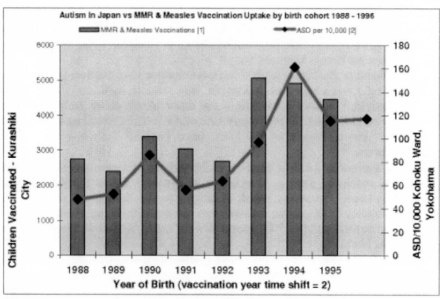

This is a comparison of Measles and MMR vaccination uptake in Kurashiki City [1] with ASD rates in a district of Yokohama [2]. The close correspondence indicates this is unlikely to be coincidental. NB 1993 births cohort vaccine uptake blue bar is unadjusted. It represents 114% vaccine uptake compared to birth rate and requires adjustment down. The uptake indicates catch-up vaccinations in 1995/6 for those born 1993/4. ([1] Terada [2] Honda/Rutter).

In 2009 the autism rate for boys in the United States was 1:96. In the UK, on March 21, 2009, a Cambridge University study showed 1 in 48 British boys has an autistic condition. This is already costing the UK £28 million per annum.[137]

In June, 2009, just months after the US Court of Federal Claims rejection of the claim that the MMR vaccine causes autism, data from formal peer-refereed medical papers was published that showed vaccines caused autism in Japanese children.[138] The number of Japanese children developing autism rose and fell in direct proportion to the number of children vaccinated each year. There is no reason to suppose that these statistics are different everywhere that MMR is given.

In June 2009, a measles outbreak in Wales set the health minister in a tizzy, so much so that she tried to make MMR a mandatory requirement for Welsh kids going to school. A physician is quoted in one UK newspaper as saying: "One in 500 children with measles dies", a statement that is clearly not supported by statistics. But because he has MD after his name, people no doubt believed him. I simply can't believe the fuss now made over measles in a time when 1:48 boys in the UK have autism. My generation all had measles and are no worse off for it.

---

[137] Daily Mail, UK, March 20, 2009
[138] http://childhealthsafety.wordpress.com/2009/06/03/japvaxautism/

One researcher with an MD after his name is Andrew Moulden, MD, Ph.D. His expertise is in neurobehavioral assessments of acquired brain and behavioral disorders. He has concluded that, because there is an influx of white blood cells when toxins are injected into the body, these clog up the smallest blood vessels, the capillaries, and thus impair the blood flow to various organs. He thus deduces that it is not the toxins that are causing the damage but the body's response to them. He holds that the impaired blood flow causes damage to the tissues in all organs but specifically in the brain so that "mini strokes" are the result and cause autism, and other neurodevelopment disorders. Moulden demonstrates the effect of these mini strokes on children with autism by comparing photographs of their eyes prior to vaccination with their eyes after vaccination. Apparently eye changes are one of the signs of a stroke. The changes are pronounced; examples can be seen on his website.[139]

Moulden says of vaccination, "By steadfastly chasing the "more profit and sales is better at any cost" lure of capitalism's "get rich" and "don't stop if it makes money" mentality, we have single handedly wiped out a generation of children, and the hopes and dreams of: 1 child in 87(autism), 15% of children with attention deficit disorders, 1 child in 6 with specific learning disabilities, 1 child in 9 with asthma, 1 child in 450 with insulin dependent diabetes, 1-2% of infants with sudden infant death, 250,000 military veterans from the Gulf War with chronic illness, and 40,000 dead(even among those who were never deployed overseas).

"And now the world is gearing up for medical martial law, and a global vaccination program for Avian flu, or some enigmatic "Spanish flu-Avian flu" hybrid.

"Whatever the "global infectious disease health crises" that confronts us now, we are in a bind, and we have put ourselves there on our own. Some are going to die of infectious diseases. Many are going to die of vaccinations or experience a plethora of chronic and obscure "ailments" from vaccinations. The addition of adjuvant to vaccines (e.g. aluminum, squalene, liposomes etc.). in an attempt to enhance and prolong the immunological challenge in the body, as it turns out, has been the single most dreadful thing man has ever done to himself, and each other."[140]

One of my favourite contentious authors is the late paediatrician, Robert Mendelsohn. In his article, "The medical time bomb of immunization against disease" he says, "I know as I write about the dangers of mass immunisation, that it is a concept that you may find difficult to accept. Immunizations have been so artfully and aggressively marketed that most parents believe them to be the "miracle" that has eliminated many once-feared diseases. Consequently, for anyone to oppose them borders on the foolhardy. For a paediatrician to attack what

---

[139] http://brainguardmd.com/
[140] http://www.curezone.com

has become the "bread and butter" of paediatric practice is equivalent to a priest's denying the infallibility of the pope."[141]

Later in the article he says, "There is a growing suspicion that immunization against relatively harmless childhood diseases may be responsible for the dramatic increase in auto-immune diseases since mass inoculations were introduced. These are fearful diseases such as cancer, leukemia, rheumatoid arthritis, multiple sclerosis, Lou Gehrig's disease, lupus erythematosus, and the Guillain-Barré syndrome. An auto-immune disease can be explained simply as one in which the body's defence mechanisms cannot distinguish between foreign invaders and ordinary body tissues, with the consequence that the body begins to destroy itself. Have we traded mumps and measles for cancer and leukemia?"

The MMR vaccine contains a 'live' measles virus. Dr. Moskowitz, from Harvard believes live viruses can lead to auto-immune diseases.[142] He posits that viruses in vaccines can attach part of their genes to the genes of the host cell. They can then remain latent for years but the presence of this foreign material "sets the stage for their unpredictable provocation of various auto-immune phenomena such as herpes, shingles, wart, tumors – both benign and malignant – and diseases of the central nervous system, such as varied forms of paralysis and inflammation of the brain."

Such diseases of the nervous system include cerebral palsy. All countries with intensive or mandatory vaccination of infants have experienced a 400% increase in the incidence of cerebral palsy in the last 50 years.[143]

When I was a child the word "allergy" was unheard of. A few people suffered from hay fever in the summer but all children could drink milk, eat nuts and consume bread without any ill effects. Indeed, a child who could not would probably not have survived WWII and its attendant food restrictions. Nowadays, nearly 5 million children in the US suffer from asthma and of those, 50-80% develop symptoms before the age of five years. The annual cost of treating children with asthma is estimated to be $1.9 billion.[144] Several clinical studies have shown an association between vaccination and asthma. For example, in 1994, Dr. Odent and colleagues found that children who received pertussis vaccine had a 5.43 greater chance of developing asthma than unvaccinated children. They also had twice as many ear infections.[145]

---

[141] Mendelsohn, R. The Medical Time Bomb of Immunization Against Disease. www.whale.to/vaccines/mendelsophn.html

[142] Obomsawin, R. Immunization. A report prepared for Canadian International Development Agency, 1992

[143] Scheibner, V. *Vaccination: 100 Years of Orthodox Research Shows that Vaccination Represents a Medical Assault on the Immune System.* New Atlantean Press, New Mexico, 1993

[144] Cave, S. & Mitchell, D. *What Your Doctor May Not Tell You About Children's Vaccinations.* Warner Books, 2001

[145] Golden, I. *Vaccination? A Review of Risks and Alternatives.* Australia, 1994

There is another side-effect of vaccination that I have not seen described in the literature. The topic of vaccination produces a paralysis of the critical faculties, a condition I have termed "Vaccimania." This is an affliction of the mind that is characterised by the following signs and symptoms:

- An unalterable belief that vaccination prevents disease, accompanied by disbelief, even anger, when confronted with evidence to the contrary.
- A willingness to allow authority figures to inject live viruses and toxins into one's body.
- Fear; fear of disease, fear of microbes and fear of not following the herd.
- An attitude that cannot tolerate the least discomfort in a child but is willing to risk death, leukaemia, autism and other profound conditions instead.
- A touching faith in a pharmaceutically controlled medical profession.
- A willingness to shoot the messenger.
- A suspension of common sense.
- In physicians and nurses, a denial that convulsions or any other adverse effects have anything to do with vaccination.
- A belief that we must "wage war" against time-limited, generally harmless infections, using huge resources but nevertheless allow chronic diseases to flourish.

Galloping Vaccimania occurred in 2004 when the US experienced a flu vaccine shortage and the following events occurred:

- A number of states and the US capital district threatened doctors and nurses with fines or even jail time if they gave flu vaccines to healthy people.
- One elderly woman died after standing in line for a flu shot at a grocery store in northern California for FIVE HOURS! With nowhere to sit, the 79-year-old woman fell as she walked to find shade, hitting her head on the pavement, and later died.
- The town of Bloomfield, N.J. held a lottery to find out who would receive one of the city's estimated 300 flu vaccines.
- In some cases, physicians were even taking verbal threats from patients. One particularly incensed patient blamed a Nebraska doctor for not being able to get a flu shot, and hoped she'd be happy "when I get sick and die because it will be your fault."
- Some 600 doses of vaccine were stolen from a paediatrician's office in Aurora, Colo.
- Price-gouging in Kansas lifted the price of a 10-dose vial from $80 to $600.[146]

---

[146] Mercola, J. Missing the Flu Diagnosis in Kids Just Another Excuse for a Vaccine. www.mercola.com

There are many conditions that are named after the first person to describe them; for example, Karposi's sarcoma, Addison's disease, Koplik's spots. And now … Craig's Vaccimania!

I wonder if this new condition will be described in the DSM (Diagnostic and Statistical Manual of Mental Disorders). In addition to signs and symptoms this manual lists known causes, statistics in terms of gender, age at onset and prognosis as well as research concerning optimal treatment approaches.

Perhaps I should approach a drug company for funding to support research into this condition. Maybe I can develop a vaccine against Vaccimania. Now wouldn't that be a breakthrough?

*   *   *

The 2206 edition of the Encylopaedia Universia lists the following entries:

Vaccine: A mixture of live or dead viruses or bacteria grown on infected animal tissue and suspended in toxic substances such as formaldehyde. Prior to the advent of energetic medicine people thought that the injection of this mixture into the bloodstream would prevent infectious disease.

Vaccination: The practice of injecting a vaccine into people, particularly children, as an infectious disease preventative. Its use was widespread for about 150 years until catastrophic epidemics of chronic diseases such as cancer, leukaemia, autism and behavioural problems, shown to be the result of vaccination, put an end to the practice.

Vaccimania: A syndrome, first described by Dr. Jennifer Craig in 2006, that affected billions of people. Propaganda, originating from the pharmaceutical industry and promoted by governments and the media, was successful in making people believe in the magical powers of vaccination.

*   *   *

Chapter 10

Legalities

"The law supposes that your wife acts under your direction," Mr. Brownlow said to Mr. Bumble in *Oliver Twist*. "If the law supposes that," said Mr. Bumble, squeezing his hat emphatically in both hands, "the law is an ass – an idiot. If that's the eye of the law, the law's a bachelor, and his eye may be opened by experience – by experience."

I tended to agree with Mr. Bumble that the law is an ass after I read the Stella Awards that are named after the woman who sued McDonalds because the coffee was hot. She won. The 2005 Stella Award winner was Mary Ubaudi of Madison County, Ill. who was a passenger in a car that crashed. She put most of the blame on Mazda Motors, who made the car she was riding in. She demanded "in excess of $150,000" from the automaker, claiming it "failed to provide instructions regarding the safe and proper use of a seatbelt." One hopes Mazda's attorneys made her swear in court that she had never before worn a seatbelt, had never flown on an airliner, and that she's too stupid to figure out how to fasten a seatbelt.

I remember reading about a British case where a man left his window open in the summer. A burglar attempted to climb through the window but the man's dog bit him. The burglar sued the man ... and won. Lawyers have a lot to answer for.

In the US childhood vaccinations are mandated by law. I recall the words of Dr. Walter Hadwen in 1896: "The very moment you take a medical prescription and you incorporate it in an Act of Parliament, and you enforce it against the will and conscience of intelligent people by fines, distraints and imprisonments, it passes beyond the confines of a purely medical question – and becomes essentially a social and political one." And that is what has happened in the US. Vaccination is a political issue, not a health one.

It's too bad that no one listened to Benjamin Rush, a Founding Father of the United States and a signer of the Declaration of Independence. He believed that Americans should enshrine the right to medical freedom in their Constitution, much as the right to freedom of religion is expressly guaranteed. Rush said, "Unless we put Medical Freedom into the Constitution, the time will come when medicine will organize into an undercover dictatorship, to restrict the art of healing to one class of men, and deny equal privilege to others, will be to constitute the

Bastille of Medical Science. All such laws are un-American and despotic and have no place in a Republic."[147] He has been proved right.

When American citizens refuse to vaccinate their children they can be denied education, including enrolment in day care, denied health insurance, denied government benefits, including food for poor children. Furthermore, parents who don't comply with vaccination laws have been charged with child medical neglect and threatened with having their children taken from them.

Is this public health practice? One of the basic tenets of medical and nursing practice is informed consent. How can doctors and public health nurses ethically subscribe to forced vaccination policies? Nurses also value the idea of individualized care. How can they rationalise mass vaccination campaigns?

When it comes to suing for vaccine damage, people are out of luck. In the US, Congress passed its *National Childhood Vaccine Injury Act* in 1986. This required all doctors who administer vaccines to report reactions to federal health officials. However the FDA estimates only 10% of doctors report such incidents.[148]

A study by Connaught Laboratories confirmed this estimate. Prior to the study period, unsolicited reports of adverse reactions occurred at the rate of 20 per million doses. When the lab supplied the vaccine with a request to report any adverse event that occurred within 30 days of vaccination, provided that it resulted in a physician visit, the rate of adverse events rose to 927 per million doses.[149]

Even this fifty-fold underreporting may be conservative. According to Dr. David Kessler, director of the FDA, "Only about one percent of serious events (adverse drug reactions) are reported to the FDA."[150] In 1998 a National Vaccine Information Center survey of New York paediatric offices found that only one doctor in 40 reports a death or an injury following vaccination.[151]

On the rare occasions when adverse reactions are reported the data can be presented in such a way that the event seems minor. For example, Sinclair quotes from a study of DPT reactions in a 1981 issue of *Paediatrics*. The article says that out of 15,752 shots only 18 children suffered serious reactions. Yet if you read carefully, each child was given five shots meaning that 3,150 children were subjects, not 15,752. Eighteen serious reactions from 3,150 children means that 1:175 experienced reactions, not 1:525.

Health and Welfare Canada provides a form to physicians and public health clinics entitled: *Report of a Vaccine-Associated Adverse Event*. They list 22 conditions that may be ticked off. I don't know how compliant Canadian health care workers are in filling out these forms but at least it acknowledges that there are adverse reactions.

---

[147] http://en.wikipedia.org/wiki/Benjamin_Rush
[148] Miller, N. *Immunization: Theory vs. Reality*. New Atlantean Press, 1995
[149] Ibid
[150] Ibid
[151] O'Shea, T. *The Sanctity of Human Blood: Vaccination I$ not Immunization*. Two Trees, San Jose, California, 2004

All professional bodies have written *Codes of Ethics and Practice Standards* that govern their members. Should a member violate the standards, that person is faced with disciplinary action that can result in their being struck off the profession's register.

At one time I was an educational consultant to the health professions. One of my most enjoyable contracts was to re-write the Practice Standards for what was then the Registered Nurses Association of British Columbia. The standards in use were non-functional, largely because nursing in the seventies and eighties was obsessed with nursing models. For example, one standard read something like, "Use a nursing model to deliver nursing care." If you don't understand what this means, take heart, neither did most practicing nurses.

The Code of Ethics for Registered Nurses in Canada is the work of the Canadian Nurses Association (CNA), whereas the College of Nursing in each province writes its own practice standards. There are three ethical standards that relate to my argument: two are about choice. One ethic reads:
*"Nurses must ensure that nursing care is provided with the person's informed consent. Nurses must recognize that persons **have the right to refuse or withdraw consent** for care or treatment at any time."*

Another ethic reads: *"Nurse must be sensitive to their position of relative power in professional relationships with persons. Nurses must also identify and minimize (and discuss with the health team) **sources of coercion**."* (My emphasis.)

Any nurse who tells a parent that she is putting other children at risk by choosing not to vaccinate her child, and I have heard of nurses who do that, is violating her ethical standards.

In the US, vaccinations are mandated by the government. The American Nurses Association's Standards for public health nurses (PHN) include: "The PHN participates in the application of public health laws, regulations and policies ... and "Assists with implementing penalties for non-compliance of laws, regulations and policies." As their Code of Ethics states, "the concept of informed choice is fundamental to the delivery of health care," American nurses are faced with conflicting directives.

A third ethic of the CNA is: *"Nurses must base their practice on relevant research findings and acquire new skills and knowledge in their area of practice throughout their career."* How cognizant are public health nurses in Canada of the research demonstrating vaccine damage? How can they believe the myth that vaccines got rid of smallpox?

In BC, the standard about Consent includes, "Nurses have legal and ethical obligations regarding client consent for proposed care, treatment and research." One of the conditions for consent is "the client or substitute decision-maker is adequately informed." Parents taking their children to public health clinics for vaccinations are not required to sign a consent form. Why not? You must sign a consent form to even set foot in an emergency room before anyone can examine you. Why not for injecting a child? Just telling a parent that adverse effects are rare is simply not good enough and it is hardly informed consent. I have designed a form for parents to sign prior to their child's vaccination. It lists the 22 conditions from the Health and Welfare Canada Adverse Event form.

Form 678234A,06
CONSENT FOR VACCINATION

I _____ certify that I understand the following information before consenting to have my child(ren), name(s) _____ _____vaccinated
(Please place a tick beside each statement to indicate understanding).
__ Vaccination does not guarantee that your child will not contract the disease.
Any of the following adverse reactions may occur as the result of vaccination:
__ Fever: three classes -- >40.5 C, 39-40.5C or not recorded.
__ Infective abscess at injection site
__ Sterile abscess at injection site
__ Severe pain or severe swelling at injection site
__ Adenopathy (enlarged glands)
__ Allergic reaction
__ Rashes
__ Anaphylaxis (collapse)
__ Hypotonic-Hyporesponsive episode/excessive somnolence (not responding)
__ Arthralgia/arthritis
__ Severe vomiting and/or diarrhea
__ Screaming episode/persistent crying
__ Convulsion/seizure
__ Encephalopathy
__ Meningitis and/or encephalitis
__ Anaesthesia/paraesthesia (numbness)
__ Paralysis
__ Guillain-Barré Syndrom
__ Subacute sclerosing panencephalitis (SSPE) (infection of central nervous system)
__ Parotitis (swollen parotid glands)
__ Orchitis (swollen testicles)
__ Thrombocytopenia (decrease in blood platelets)
__ Death

Signed _____
Date _____

But if I present this consent form to the CNA I suspect I will get the same response I received from the Night Sisters fifty years ago

The National Vaccine Injury Compensation Program (VICP) Fact Sheet of the US states: "In the early 1980s, reports of harmful side effects following the DTP (diphtheria, tetanus, pertussis) vaccine posed major liability concerns for vaccine companies and health care providers, and caused many to question the safety of the DTP vaccine. Parents began filing many more lawsuits against vaccine companies and health care providers. Vaccination rates among children began to fall and many companies that develop and produce vaccines decided to leave the marketplace, creating significant vaccine shortages and a real threat to the Nation's health."

Reading this I am struck by how the emphasis is on the "major liability concerns for vaccine companies." Where is the concern for the damaged children, the ruined lives and the devastated family? Where is the reflection that the risks might outweigh any supposed benefits? Where are the physicians who swore that first they would do no harm? Where is the reassessment of the whole idea of mass vaccination? The Nation's health seemed to be improving without vaccines in the first place so what is the "real threat"?

The fact sheet goes on: "Congress created the VICP (Vaccine Injury Compensation Program) to ensure an adequate supply of vaccines, stabilize vaccine costs, and establish and maintain an accessible and efficient forum for individuals thought to be injured by childhood vaccines. The VICP, which went into effect on October 1, 1988, is a no-fault alternative to the traditional tort system for resolving vaccine injury claims, whether the vaccine is administered in the public or private sector. Since its inception, the VICP has been a key component in **stabilizing the U.S. vaccine market** by providing liability protection to both vaccine companies and health care providers, by encouraging research and development of new and safer vaccines, and by providing for a more streamlined and "less adversarial" alternative to the traditional tort system for resolving claims." (Emphasis mine.)

Once again the VICP is more concerned with protecting pharmaceutical companies than children. Only one in four vaccine injury victims who apply for compensation are granted it. The qualifying rules require that the onset of adverse symptoms must have occurred within four hours of the administration of the vaccine. Despite this severe limitation, compensatory payments up to February, 1998, totalled more than $871 million,[152] paid for out of the public purse. (Not by the pharmaceutical industry.)

Lawsuits for vaccine damage are becoming increasingly common. A law firm in England carried a major class action lawsuit for damages arising from Britain's 1994 Measles, Mumps and Rubella campaign. The firm issued a public statement: *We know of hundreds of children who were fat and well before being vaccinated, but who are now chronically ill or seriously mentally or physically disabled. Of*

---

[152] Obomsawin, R. Universal Immunization: Medical Miracle or Masterful Mirage. www.whale.to/a/obomsawin.html

some 600 cases: the most common are autism (202); serious digestive problems (110); epilepsy (97); hearing and vision problems (40); arthritis (42); behaviour and learning problems (41); ME (24) (myalgic encephalomyelitis)*; diabetes (9); paralysis (9); blood disorders (5); brain damage (3); and death (14).*[153]

On February 25, 2008, NewsTrack reported that the Japanese government is bracing for a flood of damage suits from hundreds of people who contracted Hepatitis B through mandatory childhood vaccinations. Japan no longer mandates vaccinations. On the same date, the US government quietly conceded a vaccine-autism case in the court of Federal Claims. This case caused the current uproar in the US about whether or not there is a link between vaccines and autism.

On March 3, 2008, NewsWithViews reported that French authorities are suing a US-based company, GlaxoSmithKline, and its executives in a manslaughter case. France alleges that the company failed to fully disclose side effects from an anti-Hepatitis B vaccine distributed between 1994 and 1998.

Growing awareness about the harm of vaccination has been instrumental in the formation of activist organizations such as: Australian Vaccination Network (AVN); Vaccination Risk Awareness Network (VRAN), Canada; National Vaccine Information Center (NVIC), United States; the Immunization Awareness Society, New Zealand; and The Informed Parent Group in the UK.

In September, 1997, the First International Public Conference on Vaccination was held. At this the Presenters explained the dangerous constituents of vaccines, the harm done by them and their belief that governments have withheld information about vaccine risks from the public"[154]

When I visited my brother in South Africa he took the family to the Kruger National Park. I loved every minute of it: the wonder of seeing so many animals in the wild; camping, with baboons staring at the humans behind their protective wire fences; trying to identify a few of the numerous bird species, getting boggle eyes from staring through binoculars.

The only elephant we saw was an old guy with a broken tusk standing on the road in front of us. He looked old in the way he held his body but the jagged tusk on one side and the mature, complete, pointed one on the other, lent him an air of menace. Warned at the park gates by gruesome pictures of cars damaged by elephants, we remained in the van ready for a rapid egress should he decide to charge.

I now characterise vaccination as a monolithic pachyderm – an elephant that has run amok and is causing irreparable damage. He grows larger by the year. In 2006 the US mandated 40 vaccines for children, including boosters. And there are more in the pipe line. There is even one planned for obesity. Could someone please tell me what the causative infectious agent is in obesity? I seem to have missed that information.

Perhaps there's a "B" in both.

---

[153] Ibid.
[154] Ibid.

Chapter 11

Medical Evangelism

I was making a mushroom omelette. Just as I was about to pour the beaten eggs onto the fried mushrooms, the boom of my antique brass knocker on the door of my heritage house suspended the operation. I kneed aside my border-collie, who was issuing frenzied warnings, to open the door. Two fresh-faced young men with short haircuts, dark suits, white shirts and conservative ties stood expectantly on the porch.

My first instinct was to yell, "Bugger off!" but I remembered the painted paving stone that says "Welcome" and controlled myself. Nevertheless, I adopted what I hoped was a repellent posture – narrowed eyes, tight lips and arms akimbo.

"Good morning," one young man said; the one for whom a razor was an unnecessary bathroom implement.

"Yes?" I said, coldly.

"We are here to tell you how to let light into your life."

I switched on the porch light. His composure shrunk. The other one took up the slack. "Not that sort of light," he chuckled. "The light of Jesus." Both of them put on that seraphic look that I can't abide.

The gist of my message as they hastened down the front steps was "Don't teach your grandmother how to suck eggs." I calmed myself by wondering how that phrase came about and, abandoning the omelette, went upstairs to Google it. I found this explanation by Michael Quinion.[155]

"Its meaning is clear enough: don't give needless assistance or presume to offer advice to an expert. As that prolific author, Anon, once wrote:

Teach not thy parent's mother to extract
The embryo juices of the bird by suction.
The good old lady can that feat enact,
Quite irrespective of your kind instruction.

I reflected on my hostility towards missionaries. They have always held a heroic and romantic place within the Christian imagination. Even today churches regularly collect contributions for the mission field. The reality, of course, is very

---

[155] www.worldwidewords.org

different. From its very beginnings, Christian missionaries have inflicted tremendous harm on the peoples they "witnessed" to.

Dr. Jai Maharaj writes of missionaries: "Their destruction of native cultures, and in some cases actually *causing* the deaths of these natives, can only be described as a modern *cultural and genocidal holocaust.*

"Today the number of missionaries from liberal churches is dwindling, their numbers being taken over by the fundamentalist, Pentecostal and evangelical churches. However, much like their ecclesiastical forefathers of the previous centuries, these missionaries do not believe the Africans, now largely Christians, are smart enough to keep the faith and churches going. Thus the rallying cries of the new missionaries involve "making Africa born again" or "fighting the forces of secularism" or "battling AIDS".

Is it the social or physical well being of Africans that concerns these modern day missionaries? In the late 1980s, "Armed with US$250,000 from the Southern Baptist Convention, Dr. John Goodgame, an American missionary in Uganda, launched a most unusual campaign against AIDS. Rather than using the money to provide healthcare or medicine, the money was used to purchase and distribute 100,000 *Bibles* with sheets pasted onto them giving selected Biblical passages to read. Some of these passages are predictable exhortations against adultery and other such "carnal" pleasures."[156]

The number of liberal missionaries might be dwindling but the gap is now filled with health officials under the auspices of the World Health Organization (WHO) and the United Nations Children's Fund (UNICEF). Their aim is Universal Childhood Immunization (UCI).

In 1992, the Canadian International Development Agency (CIDA) hired Dr. Raymond Obomsawin to evaluate the UCI program. His report was unacceptable to them; it carefully outlined not only the ineffectiveness of previous vaccination campaigns but also described the side-effects.

The official view historically held by the WHO is that the life-saving benefits of mass vaccination campaigns in the Developing World far outweigh any risks; that attention to risk factors and the potential for vaccine damage is impracticable and thus a non-issue.

Not everyone in the scientific community agrees with this position. Dr. George Dick, Professor Emeritus of Pathology, London University cautions:

• Before considering immunization it must be determined that the disease in question is of sufficient severity, frequency or other importance to justify immunization against it. Furthermore, if the infection is readily treatable, there is seldom justification for immunization.

• Immunization is indicated only when the classic methods of control are demonstrably impracticable or unsuccessful.

• Before any vaccine is introduced there must be good evidence that the vaccine is effective and relatively safe. Sufficient time has not yet elapsed to

---

[156] Maharaj, J. www.newsfeeds.com

predict with any certainty the durability of immunity with the live virus vaccines, which are now in common use.

• The best type of active immunization follows a clinical or subclinical natural infection. With many diseases this often gives lifelong protection at little or no cost to the individual or the community.

• The pre-immunization decline in infectious diseases should make one careful in attributing changes in the epidemiology of some diseases to the result of a specific treatment or immunization.[157]

These are the views of Western people. What do Africans think? Kihura Nkuba, which means "one who handcuffs lightning and puts thunder in jail", founded the Greater African Radio and is president of the East African World Broadcasters Association. In 1997 he spoke at the Third International Public Conference on Vaccination about the repeated, forced live oral polio vaccination campaign conducted by WHO and UNICEF in his country. He had researched the polio vaccines and, as a broadcaster, was able to relate to his people what he had found out. Here are some extracts from his speech:

"In Africa polio does not kill anybody and they say it's very rare to catch. It's really very rare to get paralytic polio. They say it's in very rare circumstances, so what is it that is killing people in Africa? Malaria. Every five seconds a child is dying of malaria in Africa. Now to get the dose of life-saving anti-malaria is about $5 but there is no government to give anti-malaria. When somebody gets malaria, if they have no money they even die. So the question I was asking and many people were asking was "If you really want to help children, why begin with a disease that they don't have? Why not look for something that is killing them and save them from what is killing them?

"I discovered that really the whole concept of vaccination is like getting a disease, putting it in an undiseased person to cure a disease that person hasn't got. It's like if you have an army and it's fighting an enemy, and then you bring the enemy into the barracks just to see if the soldiers can defend themselves should an enemy surprise them. I mean, you don't do such things in a war. And then I started asking myself-- humanity has lived in Africa for 5.5 million years from the stage of Australopithecines to Homo sapiens. Polio vaccination in Uganda started in 1963. So if we were all to die of polio like the Minister of Health was telling us, we would have died by 1963 and it would have been 'case closed'. There would have been nobody to vaccinate. So the fact that we have survived 5.5 million years without polio vaccination shows that people can survive without it.

"So I was told by this preacher that when the government introduced the National Immunization Days in 1997, most of the children after vaccination started dying. The preacher told me that they had so much death that his cassock, that he wears to go and conduct the burial ceremony, got old. He said "I buried the children and my cassock got old."

---

[157] Obomsawin R. Universal Immunization: Medical Miracle or Masterful Mirage. www.whale.to/a/obomsawin.html

This is the program that well-intentioned people, like Rotary Club International, are supporting. By February 2005, clubs around the world had raised over $100,275 *million* dollars for the polio eradication campaign.

Needless to say, Kihura Nkuba, like all whistle-blowers, is wanted by the police. Who puts the police up to this form of harassment? Who pays? Who is benefiting by selling to Africa live polio vaccine, not used in the West because it causes polio?

The following are unedited excerpts from an article published in 2003 by the Pan Africanist Congress, an African political party:

While the Uganda police is hunting for Kihura Nkuba to question him for his remarks against vaccination, the 15th of October was the day of reckoning for the Uganda Ministry of Health and their erstwhile partners the so-called big three the World Health Organization, UNICEF and the USAID.

It was day when their massive immunization campaign was to be judged, when attendances expected to be over 100% were expected. The government had indeed done the unthinkable, it began by extending the immunizing age to a shocking fifteen years, then they decreed that all parents have to take their children for immunization regardless of their health status, they threatened those who would resist immunization with imprisonment, young and old male and female.

The Minister without Portfolio and National Political Commissar Crispus Kiyonga, himself a medical doctor and former health minister, directed the police to arrest anybody thought to be sabotaging the exercise, the minister of health, army brigadier Jim Muhwezi, with no public health background, the minister of information Nsaba Buturo who has probably never even looked at a vaccine insert, all directed the police to arrest all the parents or even children that resisted vaccination.

The small beautiful country called Uganda, spent nine million of its meagre resources marketing this European product (the money spent would have build 120,000 protected water springs, giving 30% of the country access to clean water, it would have built ten ultra modern research centers looking at, for example, pests that are threatening the banana crop, but government chose European imposed priorities.

The health official, traveling in their full option four wheel drive jeeps (yours for only $US70,000), adorning business suits of the best German design and being watered by the delights of American coca cola, have slept in every good hotel in Uganda helping the poor get the message of immunization.

Everybody in Africa knows that once you have natural measles and you recover from it, and almost everybody recovers and people have natural herbs to treat measles, measles will never come again. Indeed the elders in Africa scratched their head trying to remember when evil spirit could have engineered measles to appear second time in a victim. But the government and the wisdom monopolists of the World health organization that turned a blind eye to cigarettes and promoted formula milk not too long ago, are especially telling those who have natural immunity to go and get their fair share of these purified measles viruses.

The local councillors are not given as much as the district councillors, whose cut of the vaccine windfall is only surpassed by those of the big shots at the ministry headquarters. A notorious councillor from Bushenyi District, the district local council speaker, Odo Tayebwa, moves from house to house, dragging children hidden underneath their beds to be vaccinated at gun point. Odo Tayebwa says he is happy doing God's work.

The propaganda which would make Gobbles look like a senior saint, says that the tests were carefully carried by the World Health Organizations, most of whose doctors are seconded to drug manufactures and the UNICEF which represents the interest of European big business.

"We are doing things to our children that buffalos would never dream of doing to their calves". Yet on the day of vaccination itself, the students whom they had targeted at school stayed at home, mothers hid their children in the bush, others were hidden under the bed. In most parts of the country, particularly western and central Uganda, areas covered by Greater African Radio, the immunizers sat in classrooms without children as the boxes that contained the vaccines sweated in the chocking sun. The immunizers wore t-shirts bearing the words "kick measles out of Uganda" and gave out tops bearing the same message and plenty of American soft drinks.

What they did not see were anxious parents, or even children. At neighbouring schools in Western Uganda, learners cut the wire mesh surrounding their schools and jumped to safety, some swearing that they had better quit school than take the measles live vaccine. Some parents thought that this was polio vaccine disguised as measles.

The enthusiasm of government to give vaccines to a people to whom it normally gives nothing was seen as very suspicious.

Forcing them to take a vaccine against a disease they know to be harmless and which they know how to cure was seen as the action of a government hell bent on killing its own population for the benefit of the commanding "whiteworld." All village people know that once you have recovered from measles you will never catch it again, but here they were telling people to vaccinate even those who have recovered from measles.

In other villages police armed to the teeth moved from house to house searching for children to immunize. Peasants pressed for time to plant their crops, have now got to spend five to ten days in hiding.

As for Kihura Nkuba, he says if the government can increase their income, their sanitation, their education, then he would be prepared to negotiate. The criminal investigation department of the Uganda police is looking for Kihura Nkuba for questioning regarding his remarks he made against measles. They are blamed for poor results. The government has put a brave face on the whole exercise saying the result achieved showed that 70% had received measles. Otherwise the poor farmers of Uganda have decided to defy their government again. They have not trust their doctors and have given thumbs down to the WHO, USAID and UNICEF. In so doing however they have harvested a cup of bitterness. I am sure that soon the World Health Organization will find something wrong with black skin and a mandatory vaccine should be in existence somewhere to help us get rid of it.

*   *   *

On another continent, down under, Aboriginal parents also had to hide their children from the vaccarazo. Dr. Archie Kalokerinos describes how many of the "Aboriginal mothers, when they saw the health team coming, would grab their babies and flee into the scrub. Mainly because they could count. They knew what would happen every time the doctors came around with their needles."[158] Dr. Kalokerinos worked with Australian Aboriginals for many years and wrote about his experiences in *Every Second Child.*[159] He found out that the huge death rate among Aboriginal infants was largely due to Vitamin C deficiency and otitis media, (ear infection).

After a period in the United States, Kalokerinos returned to Australia and was asked to look into why the infant death rate in the Northern Territory had doubled in 1970 and was even higher in the first six months of 1971. For weeks and months he thought about it but the answer did not come to him. He asked himself what had changed in the Territory? "Then suddenly it clicked. 'We have stepped up the immunisation campaigns,' Ralph (my colleague), had said. My God! I had known for years that they could be dangerous, but had I underestimated this? Of course I had. There was no need to go to Alice Springs. I knew. A health team would sweep into an area, line up all the Aboriginal babies and infants and immunise them. There would be no examination, no taking of case histories, no checking on dietary deficiencies. Most infants would have colds. No wonder they died. Some would die within hours from acute Vitamin C deficiency precipitated by the immunisation. Others would suffer immunological insults and die later from 'pneumonia', 'gastroenteritis' or 'malnutrition'. If some babies and infants survived, they would be lined up again. Then there would be booster doses, shots for measles, polio and even T.B. Little wonder they died. The wonder is that any survived."

No one would listen to Kalokerinos. Indeed, he was treated with hostility. He knew that supplementing infants would result, in Alice Springs anyway, in halving the death rate. Finally, he sent registered letters to two Commonwealth experts asking for an immediate investigation and hinting that, should he be ignored and his observations proved correct, he would take legal action. This worked. He was granted research facilities that subsequently supported his observations.

In 2006, UNICEF's total income was $1.969 billion. Of this 34% is spent on early childhood education, 21% on the education of girls and 22% on vaccination. The report on their website does not mention any spending on clean water and sanitation. Merck & Co., a large producer of the world's vaccines, supports UNICEF with in-kind donations.[160]

---

[158] Sinclair, I. *Vaccination: The "Hidden" Facts. Australia,* 1992
[159] Kalokerinos, A. *Every Second Child.* Nelson, Ltd. Australia. 1974
[160] Whitney, MT. Merck set up offshore accounts to avoid U.S. taxes. NewsTarget.com, February, 2007

According to an article in the *Atlanta Journal Constitution* of September 24, 2004, the World Health Organization admits that third world vaccination programs cause nearly 23 million chronic disease infections each year. "Worldwide, the 16 billion injections administered either for vaccines or drugs in the developing world each year cause an estimated 21,000,000 cases of Hepatitis B, 2,000,000 cases of Hepatitis C, and 260,000 cases of HIV, according to the WHO," wrote David Wahlberg for the *Constitution*.

Although the WHO admits its mass vaccination programs are causing epidemics of diseases that are no less serious than the ones third world populations are being vaccinated against, it believes that the risk of infection arises from the needles used, not from the toxic vaccines.[161]

---

[161] *VRAN Newsletter*, Winter 2005

Chapter 12

Theories

Five consultants "owned" beds on my ward when I was a ward sister at Leeds Infirmary in the early sixties. Each had his quirks and foibles that I learned to tolerate and even respect. Dr. Garland, a neurologist, appeared for his rounds dressed in a morning suit of striped trousers, grey waistcoat (vest) and black jacket. The jacket always sported a carnation, earning him the nickname of 'Pansy Garland'.

Then there was Dr. Telling, an internist. Normally calm and courteous he could become incensed by some unpredictable happening that would ignite a spectacular display of temper. Once everyone around him, including the patients, was thoroughly alarmed, he settled down, as suddenly as he had erupted, into his usual smooth self.

One day he found one of his patients being "barrier-nursed". When someone was infectious we drew their curtains around their bed and could only enter the isolation cubicle wearing gowns, masks and gloves. On exiting we took off the gowns and scrubbed our hands. Dr. Telling obviously thought the whole system was ridiculous. When he saw that this was how we were treating one of his patients, he bounced down the ward like a crazed tap dancer, stomping on the floor and shouting, "There's one", stomp, "There's another", stomp, "There's one with teeth. Gotcha".

The scene was unforgettable; a senior consultant peering down at the floor, bald pate gleaming, shiny black shoe stamping on the wooden floor. An unusual silence settled on the ward as patients sat up in their beds wide-eyed with amazement. Off to one side his resident and houseman stood, clearly wondering what to do. I broke into helpless laughter. He was right. To think that we could halt the spread of infection by our methods was absurd. But we tried.

Although I never discussed it with him, Dr. Telling may not have believed in the *germ theory*. I didn't even realise that the idea of infectious diseases being caused by germs was a theory. Of course diseases like tuberculosis were caused by germs. Everyone knew that. We could even name the germs: tuberculosis is caused by *mycobacterium tuberculosis*, diphtheria by *corynebacterium diptheriae* and syphilis by *treponema pallidum*.

What I didn't know at that time was the difference between *causation* and *correlation* and how often these two concepts are confused. Because two events happen simultaneously does not mean that one caused the other. For example, an increase in the stork population paralleling an increase in human birth does not mean that storks cause pregnancies.

This difference gives rise to some interesting questions. For example, do germs cause disease or are they present because of the disease? In the summer I am plagued by fruit flies. If I leave fruit out and it has slightest blemish or crack, those pesky flies swarm. However, if I cover the fruit or put it in the fridge, the flies vanish. Unbroken fruit does not attract flies; so does the *infirmity* of the fruit attract the flies?

Another "which came first?" question: recovery from infectious disease leaves one with permanent natural immunity accompanied by antibodies. But is the individual immune because of the recovery from the infection or because of the antibodies?

Modern medicine subscribed to the germ theory largely because people listened to Louis Pasteur, 1822-1895, and not to Antoine Béchamp, 1816-1908. Pasteur, a chemist, became a favourite of the French royal court and early in his career was decorated by the Emperor Napoleon. Béchamp, a physician, chemist and pharmacist, worked tirelessly as a researcher for 53 years and when he died, the *Journal Moniteur Scientifique* required eight pages to list his scientific publications.

The great scientific questions of the mid 1800s centered on fermentation; why do things grow mould, ferment or decompose? Why should milk in the larder turn sour overnight? What is living matter? How does it come into being? Can it arise spontaneously or is it always derived from pre-existing life? These questions were of more than of academic interest for both the wine and the silk industries. In the latter case, it was seeking ways of controlling a disease of silk worms.

To explore the differing views of Pasteur and Béchamp, I have used translations from their writings to recreate one of their frequent debates. They were both French of course, so their dialogue cannot be verbatim here. A particularly useful reference is Douglas Hume's *Bechamp or Pasteur: a Lost Chapter in the History of Biology* first published in 1922 and reprinted recently.[162] Douglas Hume was a woman but used a male name in order to be published.

*   *   *

Two bearded men stand face to face in a laboratory office that is simply furnished with bookcases and a desk. Louis Pasteur is dressed in a dark suit with a velvet bow tie. Dr. Antoine Béchamp, whose office they occupy, is wearing a stained lab coat over his clothes.

Pasteur. *Non, non. Diseases arise from micro-organisms outside the body. They are in the air, in the soil, everywhere.*

Béchamp. *Tiny organisms, that I call microzyma, are present in the tissues and blood of all living organisms where they are normally quiescent and harmless. When the welfare of the body is threatened, the microzyma change into bacteria. These immediately go to work to rid the body of this harmful material. When they*

---

[162] Hume, D. *Bechamp or Pasteur: a Lost Chapter in the History of Biology.* Kessinger Publishing, 1922

have completed the task of consuming it, they immediately revert to the microzyma stage.

Pasteur. Non, non, the function of micro-organisms is constant. They are always the same shape and colour.

Béchamp. I beg your pardon, but micro-organisms change their shapes and colours to reflect the medium. This I have observed with a microscope.

Pasteur. Micro-organisms cause disease. Every disease is associated with a particular organism.

Béchamp. Non. Every disease is associated with a particular condition. For example, lack of a necessary nutrient.

Pasteur. Non, non, micro-organisms are the primary causal agent.

Béchamp. Micro-organisms only become pathogenic as the condition of the host deteriorates. Therefore, the condition of the host is the causal agent.

Pasteur. Mon ami, disease can strike anyone at any time.

Béchamp. Only when they live in unhealthy conditions or the body is in an unhealthy state.

Pasteur. To prevent disease we have to build defences, such as the use of vaccines and serums.

Béchamp. We have to create health in order to prevent disease. As bacteria do not cause disease, it follows that serums and vaccines can neither prevent nor cure. Indeed, the most serious disorders may be provoked by the injection of living organisms into the blood, into a medium not intended for them. Such injections may provoke redoubtable manifestations of the gravest morbid phenomena.

*   *   *

Louis Pasteur is said to have declared on his death bed, "Béchamp was right; the microbe is nothing; the terrain is everything."[163] But it was too late – the germ theory became the ruling medical paradigm.

The "Germ Theory" proposes that germs, viruses or bacteria, cause disease. Germs are the enemy and we must fight them. This paradigm uses war metaphors; perhaps in deference to Napoleon. For example when a person becomes ill the body has been attacked; it is an invasion from outside. We say "he won his battle against cancer", we wage war against AIDS, we fight pneumonia. Much research focuses on finding the pill to kill the invading germs. If some innocent children lose their lives as a result of the weapons deployed, then that is the cost of war. Unfortunate, yes, but sacrifices must be made if we are to win the war against disease.

One of the problems with the germ theory is that it allows governments to dismiss social and economic problems as the cause of disease, for it is much easier to blame an unseen invader rather than the squalor in which some people live. Yet evidence persists that the best indicator of health is income.[164]

---

[163] Bird, C. To Be Or Not To Be? 150 Years of Hidden Knowledge. *Nexus* magazine, April 1992

[164] Evans, RG, Barer, ML, Marmor, TR. *Why Are Some People Healthy and Others Not?* Aldine de Gruyter, New York, 1994

Because we have adopted the perception that germs cause disease, medicine became the agency charged with killing these. This in turn fostered an unhealthy relationship between the medical community and individuals. Individuals abrogate responsibility for their own health because essentially they are led to believe that there is nothing they can themselves do to stop an attack. The idea is missing that a healthy unvaccinated immune system is naturally designed to combat disease and so is the idea that keeping the immune system healthy is the best way to prevent disease and that this is not achieved by invading it with toxins, supposedly to produce antibodies.

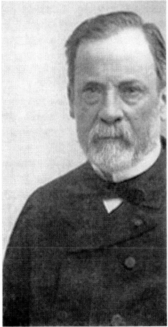

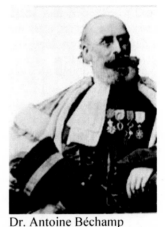

Dr. Antoine Béchamp
Physician, chemist and pharmacist
Master of Pharmacy, Doctor of Science
Doctor of Medicine, Professor of Medical Chemistry and Pharmacy at Montpellier, Fellow and Professor of Physics and Toxicology — Strasbourg Higher School of Pharmacy, Professor of Chemistry at Strasbourg, Professor of Biological Chemistry and Dean of Faculty of Medicine of Lille, Chevalier of the Legion of Honour — Commander of the Rose of Brazil

Louis Pasteur
Chemist
Friend of Napoleon

Scientists have known, at least since 2000, that the primitive concept of simply inducing antibodies does not produce immunity. The immune system is much more complex than they thought. How does the body protect itself against infection? What are the defences?[165] The first line of defence is the skin plus the fine, microscopic hairs, cilia, found in the mucous membranes of the respiratory system. Cilia move sticky material that traps undesirable substances until they can be removed by coughing or by blowing the nose. The lymphatic system comes into play along with the tonsils. In more serious cases, the process of destroying, digesting and discharging foreign proteins, antigens, from the body is known as the 'acute inflammatory response' and it is usually accompanied by fever, pain, malaise, discharges such as mucous and swollen glands and tonsils.

Tonsils are the defensive outposts of the respiratory system and their inflammation is an indication that they are working hard. I had my tonsils routinely removed when I was four years old. It was an outpatient procedure and children were sent home immediately they recovered from the anaesthetic. All I remember is my mother being unusually solicitous and a black mask being held over my face. Now I am amazed at the cavalier way an essential part of my immune system was whipped out simply because Medicine at that time did not understand why tonsils were there.

Another line of defence consists of colonies of friendly bacteria in the deeper recesses of the body such as the vagina and the bowel. These can produce antibiotic secretions that discourage unwanted bacteria and maintain an optimum acidity level wherein unfriendly bacteria cannot flourish.

Leon Chaitow, a practising naturopath, osteopath and acupuncturist, explains that there are two distinct biological defence systems: one the *immunological defence system* and the other, the much neglected *chemical defence system*. The latter includes blood, which, if healthy, is bacteriostatic in that it can immobilize bacterial invasion through its chemistry. However, blood chemistry is dependent upon adequate nutrition, particularly Vitamin C. The immunological defence system is the last line of defence after the skin and chemical factors have failed to repel invaders. It also requires adequate nutrition in order to function. [166]

Dr. Philip Incao[167] explains that in recent years scientists have learned more about the human immune system, including that it is composed of two branches: the cellular immune system (Th1 function) and the humoral immune system (Th2 function). The Th1 function is the acute inflammatory response whereas the Th2 function primarily recognises foreign antigens and produces antibodies.

Incao compares the two functions to eating: tasting and recognising food on the one hand, (Th2) and digesting the food and eliminating waste on the other (Th1). But just as too much tasting will ruin the appetite so will too much stimulation of the humoral immune system put the Th1 – Th2 systems out of balance.

---

[165] Chaitow, L. *Vaccination and Immunization: Dangers, Delusions, Alternatives*. C.W. Daniel Company Limited, 1987
[166] Ibid.
[167] Incao, PF. Vaccination from a Clinician's Perspective. *Well Beings*, November 1988

Th 1	Cellular immune system	Acute inflammatory response	Elimination of waste
Th 2	Humoral immune system	Recognises foreign antigens. Produces antibodies	Tastes and recognises food

Incao maintains that a growing number of scientists believe that the increase in allergic and auto-immune diseases is caused by the lack of stimulation of the Th1 branch, a stimulation that used to happen when children were allowed to get measles, mumps and chicken pox for example.

Dr Rebecca Carly explains it another way. She has realized that "bypassing the mucosal aspect of the immune system by directly injecting organisms into the body leads to a corruption in the immune system itself whereby IgA is transmuted into IgE, and/or the B cells are hyperactivated to produce pathologic amounts of self-attacking antibody as well as suppression of cytotoxic T cells. These are formed when vaccine viruses combine with viruses from tissues used to culture them, or when bacteria lose their cell walls when a person takes antibiotics causing a lack of some critical antigens normally recognized by the cellular immune system. Another example is stealth adapted (mutated) cytomegaloviruses which arose from African green monkey (simian) kidney cells when they were used to culture polio virus for live polio virus vaccines. Thus, not only was the vaccinee inoculated with polio, but with the cytomegalovirus – and many other monkey viruses as well.

"The mechanism by which the immune system is corrupted can best be realized when you understand that the two poles of the immune system (the cellular and humoral mechanisms) have a reciprocal relationship in that when the activity of one pole is increased, the other must decrease. Thus, when one is stimulated, the other is inhibited. Since vaccines activate the B cells to secrete antibody, the cytotoxic (killer) T cells are subsequently suppressed.

"In fact, the prevention of a disease via vaccination is, in reality, an inability to expel organisms due to the suppression of the cell-mediated response. Thus, rather than preventing disease, the disease is actually prevented from ever being resolved."

The idea of vaccination is to introduce a disease agent into a person's body without causing the disease. If the vaccine provoked the whole system it would cause all the symptoms of the disease. The trick is to stimulate the immune system just enough so that it makes antibodies but not enough to provoke an acute inflammatory response. However, as we have seen, all this does is shift the Th1 – Th2 balance towards Th2, the antibody producing system and mar the functioning of the immune system for when it really needs to come into play.

A study by Dr. Alec Burton for the British Medical Council in 1950 investigated the relationship between the incidence of diphtheria and the presence of antibodies. He concluded that there was no relation whatsoever between antibody count and incidence of disease. Furthermore, Dr. Burton discovered that children born with a-gamma globulinaemia (an inability to produce antibodies) develop and recover from measles and other infectious diseases almost as quickly and spontaneously as other children.[168]

Even the Centers for Disease Control (CDC) acknowledge that *antibodies do not protect us from infection*. For example, the HiB (Haemophilus influenzae type B) vaccine insert states, "The antibody contribution to clinical protection is unknown." And a JAMA article on smallpox asserts: "Neutralizing antibodies are reported to reflect levels of protection, although this has not been validated in the field."[169]

Thus, contrary to general belief, vaccinations do not strengthen the whole immune system. Instead, as we have seen, they over-stimulate the antibody production function and simultaneously suppress the cellular immune system. Dr. Richard Moskowitz, graduate of Harvard and New York Medical School, says: "Vaccines trick the body so that it will no longer initiate a generalized inflammatory response. They thereby accomplish what the entire immune system seems to have evolved to prevent. They place the virus directly into the blood and give it access to the major immune organs and tissues without any obvious way of getting rid of it."[170] In other words, what is prevented is not the disease but the ability of our immune system to manifest, respond to and overcome the disease.

Harold Buttram (physician) and John Hoffman, (medical researcher) gathered evidence to support their hypothesis of vaccine-induced malfunction. Among their many observations is that, given the one cell-one antibody rule, once a plasma cell or a lymphocyte deals with a given antigen, it becomes inert; that is, it's out of the fight and can't respond to other attacks on the immune system. During usual childhood diseases up to seven percent of the child's immune capacity is used. However, up to 70% is used in response to routine childhood vaccinations, never to be available again.[171]

Health authorities subscribe to the theory of herd immunity. I like to do crosswords, quick crosswords that is, not the cryptic sort when the clue is so obscure that I don't understand how they arrived at the answer. I can solve straightforward clues such as, 'What is the collective term for budgerigars?' Answer: a chatter. Collective terms fascinate me – a pride of lions, a colony of beavers, a flock of birds – and I wonder how they arose.

---

[168] James, W. *Immunizations: The Reality Beyond the Myth*. Bergin & Gervey, 1988

[169] Henderson et al. Smallpox as a biological weapon: medical and public health management. *Journal of the American Medical Association*, June 9, 1999, Vol. 281 p.3132

[170] James, W. *Immunizations: The Reality Beyond the Myth*. Bergin & Gervey, 1988

[171] Obomsawin, R. Immunization: a Report for CIDA, May 1992. Buttram, Dr. Harold E. and Hoffman, John Chriss: *Vaccination and Immune Malfunction* (U.S.A., 1982) (ISBN 0-916285-36-7)

What is the collective term for humans? According to health authorities it's 'herd.' Gatherings of bison, caribou, cattle, goats and moose are all herds so perhaps health authorities think we are cloven-hoofed. Anyway, they subscribe to the theory of 'herd immunity.' This states that an entire group can be protected from infectious disease if an unproven percentage of them are vaccinated. The aim is, of course, 100 percent but, since some people cannot be vaccinated because they have, for example, an immune disorder, the authorities will settle for 95 percent. It is this theory that drives the mandated vaccination policies.

But, one of the problems with the herd immunity theory, apart from a lack of a scientific basis, is that over the years many outbreaks of disease have occurred among people who are largely vaccinated against that disease, thus disproving the theory. And it is this theory that leads vaccination advocates to tell parents who chose not to vaccinate their children that they are endangering the public.

I wish Dr. Telling was still alive; I would dearly like to know if he favoured Béchamp or Pasteur.

Chapter 13

Influenza

Last Fall, a friend who used to live in Nelson came to visit. I put the kettle on and we settled down to catch up on each other's news.

"Have you had your flu shot?" my friend, I'll call her D, asked.

"Of course not!" I said stoutly. I wondered why she didn't know about my views on vaccination and then I felt grateful for a friend who was not thoroughly tired of listening to me. My son doesn't want to know; my daughter figures she's heard it all, and my regular friends are more interested in the state of my mental health after investigating all this.

"Why not?" D asked.

"Why on earth would I put poisons in my body in an effort to prevent a condition, only 20% of which is influenza?"

"What do you mean?"

"There are many pathogens that cause respiratory illnesses and only 20% of those are due to an influenza virus."[172] I poured the tea. "I figure I'm healthy enough to withstand a bout of flu. I go to bed and drink plenty of water." D grunted and looked doubtful. I continued, "Do you know what *They* do to make a flu vaccine? *They* catch birds in Asia in the summer and isolate viruses. Then *they* take a guess as to which three viruses to put in the vaccine. So if they're wrong, like they were in 2003–2004, the vaccine does not contain the naughty virus.

"Then they grow those three viruses in fertilized eggs and add the other goodies, like mercury and antibiotics. Mercury for goodness sake. No wonder there's ten times increased chance of getting Alzheimer's if you've had a flu shot five years in a row.[173] The only blessing is that you might forget to go for it. Not only that, how much do you weigh?"

"What's my weight got to do with it?"

---

[172] Fisher, BL. The Vaccine Reaction. Special Report of the National Vaccine Information Center, Spring 2004

[173] Fudenberg, H. Speech at the NVIC International Vaccine Conference, 1977

"Most flu vaccines contain 25 micrograms of mercury per dose. The EPA allowable daily exposure is 0.1 micrograms per kilogram, which means that you must weigh 550 pounds to meet the exposure guidelines."[174]

By this time D looked as if she wanted to change the subject but I continued anyway; nothing like a captive subject when I'm on a roll. "You've gone daft in your old age, D," I said. (She's from Yorkshire too.) "Doesn't tha know a scam when tha sees one?"

"But people die from the flu," D said.

"How many?" I challenged.

"Well, I don't know, but that's what *They* tell us."

"Let's look at some stats about flu deaths. The CDC's own official records in *National Vital Statistics Reports* show that a few hundred people die from flu in an average year in the US. And most of those deaths occur in the elderly or in people with pre-existing serious illnesses. For example, in 2002, the number who died from flu was 753.[175] And what's the population of the US? The Census Bureau says it's 299,541,342. That means that 299,540,589 did not die of flu. And of the 753 who did die, 59% were people over 75 years and 75% were people over 55 years."

"It's not the cough that carried him off, it's the coffin they carried him off in," D said, obviously back to normal.

"What carries them off is pneumonia, not flu. So why don't they give a pneumonia vaccine?"

As D's mouth was full of a Kootenay Bakery cream puff she didn't reply.

"Do you know about the damage flu vaccines cause?" D just shook her head, rather longer than necessary to indicate "no". "Look at this." I pulled out an article from my Flu file.[176] "One hundred and one citations about flu vaccine damage. And from heavyweight medical journals like the *American Journal of Psychiatry.*"

"Psychiatry? Do you go nuts after a flu vaccine?"

"Delirium. Look at this – lupus erythematosus. I love those words but the disease is nasty. Rheumatic complications, thromobocytopenia and severe neutropenia. Bullous pemphigoid ..."

"What the hell's that?"

"I dunno." I reached for my ancient medical dictionary. "A chronic, usually nonfatal, bullous skin disorder seen in middle-aged or elderly persons. Let's have a look at your skin. Are you or are you not bullous?" D held her arms close to her chest. I continued to read the citations of flu vaccine damage. "Lots of Guillain-Barre. Optic neuropathy. Ocular complications."

"Ocular complications?" D looked thoughtful. "You know, I've been having a problem with red, itchy eyes."

"When did it start?"

"About two weeks after my flu shot."

---

[174] Ayoub, D. Thimerosal: Definite cause of autism. *Scoop*, March 2005
[175] Miller, NZ. Annual Flu Deaths: The Big Lie. www.thinktwice.com
[176] www.whale/to. Citations of Flu Vaccine Damage.

"That's what happens to daft buggers who believe everything Experts tell them," I said, oozing sympathy.

"Come to think of it, I know someone, a teacher, who gets pink eye after every flu shot. But she still goes for them."

"Baa, baa." I imitated a sheep. "Can't she read? Can't she research? What is it about people that they are so willing to inject noxious substances into themselves? You know, D, I don't think we've progressed as a species since the middle ages."

"Yes we have. We have toothpaste in tubes instead of in little, round tins and we have flush toilets and we have kid-proof pill containers that kids can open but I can't."

"I mean progressed in our thinking. We are as gullible as ever and common sense ain't so common any more. Another cup?"

D picked up my file and pulled out an article at random. "Ah, the coming bird flu pandemic. Now that's something to worry about."

"It's as daft as all that brou-ha-ha that went on at the turn of the century. People made fortunes convincing the public that all our systems were going to shut down and managed to sell them tanks of propane, miles of duck tape and crates of tinned food. Talk about hysteria!"

"The WHO is predicting that 30% of the world's population will die from avian flu," D said.

"And you believe that? So far, in nine years, 100 people have died. It's a real threat."

"Yes, but millions of birds have died from it and soon it will cross over to humans."

"Yeah, right. And guess what? Vaccines will save us!" I said. "Ask yourself, what is the evidence? How many birds did they test for this amazing new virus?"

"They say it's the H5NI virus."

"Sounds awesome." I pulled out an article by Tim O'Shea.[177] "This fellow says that in 2003-2004 scientists found H5NI virus in the poultry of eight Asian nations. And since most of the birds were dead, the inference is that the virus killed them. But there's no proof of that. Each bird would have to be cultured to prove that. And *They* haven't looked at any countries, Asian or otherwise, where the virus was *not* found. So maybe it's a normal virus in birds."

"Surely we can believe what the WHO tells us?" D said.

I stared at her in amazement. "Do you believe what politicians tell you? D, it's a political organization. Their whole stance is that what ails the world can be cured by one thing only – pharmaceutical drugs. Its propaganda is something else again. Let's look at their FAQ sheet on avian flu." I pulled out my copy with its highlighted sentences. "Read this. 'The current outbreaks of highly pathogenic avian influenza, which began in Asia in mid-2003, are the largest and most severe on record.' What outbreaks? They go on: 'In 1997, in the first recorded instance of

---

[177] O'Shea, T. Avian Flu: the Pandemic That Will Never Be.
www.thedoctorwithin.com

human infection with H5NI, the virus infected 18 people and killed six of them. In early 2003, the virus caused two infections.' So that's 20 people in a part of the world with 1.8 billion people. And that's the largest and most severe outbreak on record?"

"But why would the WHO tell us all this?"

"Oh, come off it, D. To sell drugs of course. The sales of Tamiflu were over $254 million in 2004 and more than $1000 million in 2005. It didn't do a damn thing but people still bought it. And you know who produces Tamiflu? Gilead Sciences. And you know who was president of Gilead Sciences and is still a major shareholder? Donald Rumsfeld, Secretary of Defence of the USA. Go figure."

"Go figure? That's not a Yorkshire expression."

"I'm Canadian now. The most hilarious thing about all this is that Tamiflu at $100 a pop, is made from a Chinese spice called Star Anise. This is also found in Garam Masala, an Indian spice."

"I'll spread some on my dinner tonight," D said.

"The latest scandal is that Baxter International was caught shipping *live avian flu viruses* mixed with vaccine material to medical distributors in 18 countries. The "mistake" was discovered by the National Microbiology lab in Canada," I said as I read a news bulletin of March 3, 2009.[178] "They were obviously trying to give this predicted pandemic a helping hand."

"It must have been an accident."

"No way, D. Baxter adheres to something called BSL3 (Biosafety Level 3), a set of laboratory safety protocols that prevent the cross-contamination of materials. No, it was intentional all right. A global bird flu pandemic would sell a lot of vaccines. Baxter put the safety of the entire human race at risk and we have hardly heard about it in the media."

D looked doubtful. "If you don't think this could happen, D, think of Enron, Exxon, Merck, DuPont, Monsanto ... need I go on? Corporations these days are ethically challenged. The people responsible should be in gaol for attempted manslaughter and the media is either corrupt, blind or stupid for not picking up on it."

I could feel my blood pressure rising so I flicked through my file and pulled out a copy of the BBC News of 2006/07/06 with a heading of "Glaxo has bird flu 'breakthrough.'" I showed it to D. "Whenever you see the word 'breakthrough', turn on your crap detector. Hear this: 'UK drugs firm GlaxoSmithKline *believes* it has developed a vaccine for the H5NI *deadly* strain of bird flu that *may* be capable of being mass produced by 2007.' Now isn't that heartening? They *believe* they have a vaccine, but they don't know. How wouldn't you know if you have a vaccine?"

"Look at this," D said, entering into the spirit of inquiry. "Bush gave $272 million to Glaxo to produce vaccines."

---

[178] www.naturalnews.com

"Now you've got the picture, D. And you know what's going to happen? Nowt. Nada. They'll give *our* money to Big Pharma and we'll never hear about bird flu pandemics again. We've been through post-9/11 smallpox, now this and next will be the bubonic plague. That one has already started. We've been warned it's broken out somewhere, I can't recall where, and then we'll be taken through the cycle."

"What cycle?"

"Media hysteria. Millions are going to die of this coming pandemic. Look at the Middle Ages. "Scientists" will predict untold miseries. Then Big Pharma will step in with new medicines and vaccines. Governments will give them the money, our money. Then the threat of plague will mysteriously disappear."

D was still looking at the BBC News article. She read, "The news of the work on a potential vaccine came as Glaxo reported its profits had risen 14% in the three months to June to US $2.4 billion." She looked up. "Good grief; 2.4 billion dollars in three months?"

I could see the light dawning and then she said, "Yes, but vaccinations did rid the world of smallpox."

"Ahhhhhhhhhhhhhhh ..." Thump.

An instructive series of events, known as the "swine flu fiasco" took place in the US in 1976. Five soldiers in Fort Dix, New Jersey became sick. A sample of a virus was sent to the CDC who identified it as a swine flu virus that they believed, incorrectly, to be the virus responsible for the 1918 flu epidemic. They sent out a worldwide pandemic alert.

The 1918 Spanish flu epidemic was reported in the 1930s by Emeritus Professor Robert E. Shope of Yale to be caused primarily by bacteria, not by a virus at all (and this in 2009 was confirmed by other scientists) but it seems that no one at CDC checked.[179]

In the 1976 incident the CDC sent a sample to Fort Detrick, a biological warfare unit, who detected an ordinary pig virus and reported there was no need for alarm. Dr. Anthony Morris of the FDA confirmed that there was nothing in the virus to distinguish it from other swine strains and not to worry.

Nevertheless, the CDC planned a mass vaccination campaign. In 1976, President Ford authorized $135 million for the campaign and by the end of November 150 million doses of vaccine had been produced. Forty million adults were vaccinated.

In the four months following vaccination, hundreds of cases of Guillain-Barré syndrome occurred with numerous deaths. Lawsuits were lodged and nearly $3 billion was paid in compensation for suspected vaccine damage.

Dr. Morris looked closely at the vaccine and reaffirmed the public's concern about its safety and effectiveness. And that was his undoing: the FDA fired him. Dr. Morris said of flu vaccines. "It's a medical rip-off... We should recognize that

---

[179] R. Shope *Journal of Experimental Medicine;* 1936 63; 669-684, also 1931 54: 361-371 and 373-485

we don't know enough about the dangers associated with flu vaccine. I believe the public should have truthful information on the basis of which they can determine whether or not to take the vaccine." He added, "I believe that, given full information, they won't take the vaccine."[180]

In 2003 the Centers for Disease Control in the 63 U.S. again became alarmed when the rate of compliance with taking a flu shot fell to 65%. Glen Nowak, Ph.D., the Associate Director for Communications at the National Immunization Program prepared a slide-tape show called "Planning for the 2004-05 Influenza Vaccination Season: A Communication Situation Analysis."[181]

Here is a synopsis of the CDC's plan:

Step 1: *Start discussing the flu at the beginning of the "immunization season."*

Posters, fliers and media campaign materials are generally mailed to public health departments and healthcare provider offices in mid-August, "planting the seeds" in the minds of patients so that they request the flu vaccine when it arrives.

Step 2: *The media will begin to make pronouncements that the "new" influenza strains anticipated this year "will be associated with severe illness and serious outcomes."*

Right on cue, the government announced on August 25, 2004, that it is "preparing for world's next big flu outbreak." A report released to the Associated Press suggests that a bad flu season could kill up to 207,000 Americans. The CDC and the Department of Human Services announced that they are jointly issuing a *"The Pandemic Influenza Response and Preparedness Plan"* which will stress "ways to speed up vaccine production, limit the spread of a super-flu, and care for the ill."

Step 3: *The build up will continue throughout the early fall, as local and national "medical experts and public health authorities publicly (e.g., via media) state concern and alarm (***by predicting dire outcomes***)–and urge influenza vaccination."*

Here's one example:

"We know we're going to have a pandemic because, historically, we're overdue for one," said Neil Pascoe, epidemiologist in the infectious disease division of the Texas Department of Health. "When it happens, it's going to be huge. It will be global, and everyone is going to be affected...it could be terribly fatal. Imagine 4 million Texans [becoming] infected, and 20 percent of them die."

Step 4: *Reports from medical experts will be used to "frame the flu season in terms [that will] motivate behavior." Language to be used includes, "very severe," "more severe than last or past years," "deadly".*

In 2004 there were 1026 messages sent via the media between September 21-28. Phrases used included, "this could be the worst flu season ever," "the flu kills

---

[180] Butler, H&P. *Just a Little Prick.* Robert Reisinger Memorial Trust, New Zealand, 2006

[181] Nowak, G. *Planning for the 2004-2005 Influenza Vaccination Season. A Communication Analysis.* CDC.

36,000 people per year" and "the flu shot is the best way to prevent the flu." Less than 175 people actually died from influenza in 2003. [182]

Steps 5: *Continue to release reports from health officials through the media that influenza is causing severe illness and/or affecting lots of people* "**helping to foster the perception** *that many people are susceptible to a bad case of influenza.*"

Step 6: *Give visible and tangible examples of the seriousness of influenza by showing pictures of ill children and affected families who are willing to come forward with their stories. "Show pictures of people being vaccinated,* **the first to motivate, the latter to reinforce."**

Step 7: *List references to, and have discussions regarding, the influenza pandemic. "Make continued reference to the importance of vaccination."*

The language used to describe Steps 5, 6, and 7 is taken directly from Nowak's presentation. This presentation should leave little doubt that the government uses the media to create hysteria, a hysteria that will increase the demand for a pharmaceutical product.

Peter Doshi, a graduate student at Harvard University, describes how, when 50 million doses of vaccine suddenly became unavailable in 2004, the CDC downgraded its portrayal of the flu to "an annoying illness" from which most people "will recover just fine." Once the vaccines started to roll back into circulation, the CDC reverted back to its fear-mongering saying such things as, "the flu is not a benign illness. Many people don't appreciate that it can result in hospitalization, and for about 36,000 people, death." As we have seen, their own records show that influenza deaths number in the hundreds, not thousands, annually. [183]

Just in case people might suffer from side-effects of this government-sponsored campaign, Congress then passed a bill that conferred blanket immunity from prosecution for vaccine-caused illness on the makers of these vaccines. If anything goes wrong, the manufacturers cannot be sued.

The *British Medical Journal* published one of the few non-pharmaceutical company sponsored studies of the flu vaccine in October 2006. The study question was, "Each year enormous effort goes into producing influenza vaccines for that specific year and delivering them to appropriate sections of the population. Is this effort justified?"

The conclusions included: 1) Evidence from systematic review shows that inactivated vaccines have little or no effect on the effects measured, i.e. efficacy, effectiveness and safety; 2) Most studies (of flu vaccines) are of poor

---

[182] Tenpenny, S. *The Flu Season Campaign Begins.* www. NMAseminars.com

[183] Doshi, P. Viral Marketing: The selling of the flu vaccine. *Harper's Magazine*, March 2006. Vol. 312, No. 1870

methodological quality and the impact of confounders is high; 3) Little comparative evidence exists on the safety of these vaccines. [184]

I had to remind myself again of the difference between efficacy and effectiveness so I consulted my wrinkly notes from courses in epidemiology. Efficacy is the extent to which a specific intervention, procedure, regimen of service produces a beneficial effect *under ideal conditions* whereas effectiveness is the extent to which a specific intervention, procedure, regimen of service, when deployed in the field, does what it is intended to do for a defined population. Unlike efficacy, effectiveness is affected by compliance, cost and other factors that get in the way. At least, that's the way epidemiologists use the terms but they are often used synonymously in the media.

A UK case-control study of the effect of influenza vaccination on elderly patients with acute respiratory illness reported in September 2007[185] that the flu vaccine did not have an effect on the number of emergency respiratory admissions. The authors stated, "Policy makers should not rely solely on influenza vaccine routinely having a large effect on winter pressures, and should focus on additional preventive strategies."

Only people suffering from severe Vaccimania will ignore the evidence and continue to fill their bodies with mercury and flu viruses. Good luck to them.

---

[184] Jefferson, T. Influenza vaccination: policy versus evidence. *British Medical Journal,* October 28, 2006
[185] www.nhs.uk/resources/?id=271182

Chapter 14

Propaganda

The tools of propaganda: *deceit, dissimulation and distraction,* are not modern inventions. [186] In the days when salesmen peddled patent medicines, elixirs and medical cure-alls, these techniques were stock in trade. However, the pharmaceutical industry, which seems to control modern medicine, has brought these techniques to new highs.

> ♫ We'll drink a drink a drink
> To Lily the Pink the Pink the Pink
> The saviour of the human race
> She invented medicinal compound
> Efficacious in every case.
> (Traditional.)

I used to sing the chorus of this song over and over again in the sixties when the Irish Rovers made it popular. Lily the Pink was Lydia Pinkham. In 1875, after her first husband went bankrupt, Lydia started probably the first widely successful business run by a woman. Lydia E. Pinkham's Vegetable Compound for "all those painful Complaints and Weaknesses so common to our best female population" was very well advertised.

However, Lydia did not invent the medicinal compound, as Joe Nickell[187] reveals in an interesting history of patent medicines. The first royal patent for a medicinal compound is unknown but the second was granted to Richard Stoughton's Elixir in 1712. By the mid-eighteenth century, when Lydia Pinkham's vegetable compound was touted, patents protected 202 proprietary medicines. Patents required full disclosure of all ingredients so not all ready-made medicines were patented. They instead had their brand name registered. Nevertheless, the term "patent medicine" has come to mean self-prescribed nostrums and cure-alls.

I have often heard the expression "snake oil salesman" but as I didn't know where it came from, I searched the internet. Snake oil has become synonymous with a quack medicine but was originally, and still is, sold in China as a remedy for joint pain. Because snake oil contains eicosapentacnic acid (EPA), an omega 3

---

[186] O'Shea, T. The Doors of Perception: Why Americans will Believe Almost Anything. www.thedoctorwithin.com
[187] Nickell, J. www.esicop.org

derivative, a known pain reliever, it is not considered a hoax in China but is widely used in traditional Chinese medicine.

True snake oil is derived from Chinese water snakes and may contain up to 4% EPA. American products on the other hand, were made from rattlesnake fats and contained barely 1/3 of the EPA of the Chinese water snakes. For this reason they were likely to have been useless and snake oil got the reputation it has.

"The medicine peddlers used a number of tricks and stunts. The larger traveling shows, employing advance men to herald their arrival, entered town with circus-like fanfare, typically with a band leading the procession of wagons. Skits and other diversions were used to attract audiences, who eventually were treated to the "Lecture" (which, when medicine shows expanded into radio, became the commercial.)"[188] The three strategies the medicine peddlers used – deceit, dissimulation and distraction – are the tools of propaganda still in use today.

Deceit: deliberate misrepresentation of fact.

Every day *BBC News* sends me headlines; one mouse click on any headline that interests me and I can read the whole article. One headline on April 3, 2006, read "First Measles Death for 14 Years." The article told me this death was of a 13-year old boy who was suffering from an "underlying lung condition" that required taking an "immunosuppressive drug." Clearly, he was seriously ill before he contracted measles. *The Lancet* (1/8/1981) says, "In the UK about 1% of people with measles are admitted to hospital and one in ten thousand die ... children who die from measles are typically those with malnutrition or some other severe current condition, who would soon die from some other cause if not from measles."

Nevertheless, the UK's Health Protection Agency (HPA) shook its finger and stated, "the case underlies the need for all parents to ensure their children are vaccinated against the disease." Accompany deceit with threat and you have powerful propaganda.

The HPA seems to have forgotten the measles outbreaks in fully vaccinated communities but more importantly it ignores the fact that measles is a mild childhood disease that did not require a vaccine in the first place. Right now a class action is in progress on behalf of 600 British children reported damaged by the measles vaccine.

To persuade people to line up their children for injections, disease must be seen as a current **threat**. Never mind the statistics; they simply muddy the water. Your children will suffer brain damage, go deaf, die from measles if they don't get their MMR shot. Those that don't are a **threat** to everyone else. **You** will be responsible for a catastrophic measles outbreak if you don't do what we say. What does this sort of deceit say about responsible journalism?

---

[188] Ibid.

Dissimulation: to pretend *not* to be something you are.

In early summer a friend and I were walking along an unpaved country road in the Kettle River valley. Stretched across our path was what looked like a five-foot tree branch. Closer examination revealed it to be a live rattlesnake lying completely straight and motionless. This is a perfect act of dissimulation.

Many organizations have been set up to deal with the health of the public. These include the World Health Organization, (WHO), Britain's HPA, the Centers for Disease Control (CDC) and the Federal Drug Administration, (FDA) of the US, and Health Canada, but it is hard to believe that they are not agents for the pharmaceutical industry. For example, *USA TODAY,* 09/25/00, analysed the financial conflicts of interest from January 1, 1998 to June 30, 1999 in 159 FDA advisory committee meetings. It found:

- 92% of the meetings had at least one member who had a financial conflict of interest.
- At 55% of advisory meetings, at least half, sometimes more, of the FDA advisers had conflicts of interest.
- Financial conflicts of interest were possessed by 92% of those attending 57 meetings where broad health issues were discussed.
- At 102 meetings discussing the approval of a drug, 33% of the experts in attendance had a financial conflict.[189]

Congressman, Dan Burton, who testified at the 2000 US Congressional hearings on vaccine safety, asked the following questions: "How confident can we be in the recommendations of the Food and Drug Administration when the chairman (of Vaccines and Related Biological Products Advisory Committee) and other individuals on their advisory committee own stock in major manufacturers of vaccines? How confident can we be in a system when the agency seems to feel that the number of experts is so few that everyone has a conflict and thus waivers must be granted? It almost appears that there is an "old boys' network" of vaccine advisors that rotate between the CDC and FDA – at times serving both simultaneously... It is important to determine if the Department of Health and Human Services has become complacent in their implementation of the legal requirement on conflicts of interest and committee management. If the law is too loose, we need to change it. If the agencies aren't doing their job, they need to be held accountable... What is at issue is not whether the researchers can be bought in

---

[189] Ellison, S. *Health Myths Exposed.* Authorhouse, 2004

the sense of quid pro quo, it is that close and remunerative collaboration with a company naturally creates goodwill on the part of the researchers and the hope that the largesse will continue... Can the FDA and the CDC really believe that scientists are more immune to self-interest than other people?"[190]

Congressman Dan Burton is not the only person with concerns about the effect of financial interests on health decisions. John Le Carré the author, stated in an interview in 2001, "Big Pharma (the industry in general) is engaged in the deliberate seduction of the medical profession, country by country, worldwide. It is spending a fortune on influencing, hiring and purchasing academic judgment to a point where, in a few years' time, if Big Pharma continues unchecked on its present happy path, unbought medical opinion will be hard to find."[191]

In Britain, GPs receive an annual bonus of more than £2,500 (approximately $5000 US) if they vaccinate 90% of two-year-olds on their lists. A spokesperson for the British Medical Association said the bonuses are used to motivate doctors to ensure local communities are properly vaccinated. If parents choose not to vaccinate their children they are likely to be struck off their doctor's list and told to find another doctor.[192] Who pays this bonus? Why is it necessary? How is it different from a bribe? Medical ethics dictate a patient's right to refuse treatment; why is this refusal an acceptable choice for all treatments except vaccination? And why can patients refuse other treatments without losing medical services?

Distraction: to draw attention away from something.

Distraction is easy to implement. The goal is to prevent the public from thinking for themselves, to persuade them to believe authority figures such as physicians and to encourage them to ostracize those who don't follow the herd. Distractions include: the release of sensational "news"; use of alarmist language such as "Thousands may die," "Deadly virus," and "Pandemic;" pictures of suffering Africans; and relentless and repetitious messages such as "vaccine-preventable disease." And the big one – the dangers of illegal drugs, which are portrayed as far more serious than legal drugs such as vaccines.

Fear-mongering is not confined to North America. Dr. Gerhard Buchwald, a German physician, says in his book, *Impfen – Das Geschäft mit der Angst* (Vaccination – A Business Based on Fear),[193] "I have lectured all over the world ... I have always had a special interest in newspapers. All of them have one thing in common, there is always some reference made to some epidemic in some part of the world. For instance, two years ago, one paper referred to a polio epidemic in Holland. For the past three years, our newspapers have commented on the diphtheria epidemic in Russia. By these means, the population is constantly

---

[190] Ibid.
[191] Ransom, S. *Wake Up to Health in the Twenty First Century.* Credence Publications, 2003
[192] Guardian Newspapers Ltd. August 29, 1999
[193] www.whale/to

threatened with epidemics and made to fear them, and the reports always conclude: "Go and get vaccinated."

Let's look at how the Centers for Disease Control (CDC) and Health Canada promote vaccination. They each have a website article, "Misconceptions about Vaccines and Facts". They certainly do have misconceptions about facts!

The preamble states, "It was over 200 years ago that Jenner was able to protect a man from the dreaded disease smallpox through vaccination." Clearly the unidentified authors have not read their history. A faulty premise can, of course, misdirect an entire enterprise as this one has done with vaccination. For example, the germ theory, first introduced in the nineteenth century, sent scientists searching for a bacterial cause of pellagra, a disease characterized by scaly skin sores, diarrhoea, inflamed mucous membranes, mental confusion and delusions. Not until 1915 was the disease recognised as a vitamin deficiency by Dr. Joseph Goldberger who observed the difference in diets of inmates in two institutions, one of which was pellagra-free and the other suffered a high incidence of the disease. Like most doctors who challenge current thinking, Goldberger was much reviled by his colleagues.[194] Later, scientists identified the deficient vitamin as niacin, Vitamin B3. It wasn't until WW2 that the medical establishment finally accepted the idea.

The myth that Jenner prevented smallpox, a premise that is easily refuted by statistics, has turned into a huge and profitable industry. The WHO reports that 12 billion injections are given across the world annually.[195] Vaccine sales are expected to reach $10 billion in 2006, up from $5.4 billion in 2001. Are the CDC and Health Canada pushers for the pharmaceutical industry?

The CDC and Health Canada's article continues with, "Since that time, through mass immunization efforts, smallpox has been eradicated from the planet." Was it Goebbels who said the bigger the lie, the more people will believe it?

The authors of this article are unknown so I cannot comment on their credentials but as Dr. Glen Dettman is a Fellow of the Institute of Science and Technology (UK), Royal Society of Health (London), Royal Microscopical Society (UK), Australian College of Biomedical Scientists, and of the International Academy of Preventive Medicine, I assume he knows what he's talking about. He says, "It is pathetic – ludicrous to say we ever vanquished smallpox with vaccines when only 10% of the population was ever vaccinated."[196]

Health Canada continues with, "Other miracles have taken place such as the elimination of polio from the Americas (a disease that 40 years ago caused paralytic illness in almost 2000 Canadians in one year) ..." This implies that

[194] Duesberg, PH. *Inventing the AIDS Virus*. Regnery Publishing, 1996
[195] Ransom, S. *Wake Up to Health in the Twenty First Century*. Credence Publications, 2003
[196] www.whale/to

everyone who got polio became paralysed. We have seen that polio is a mild disease with about 1% suffering from paralysis, not always permanent. Health Canada fails to mention how many polio cases occurred as a result of the vaccine but when you believe in miracles facts fly out of the window.

What happened when the vaccine failed to prevent the cases of paralysis was that the health authorities renamed "paralytic polio" as Acute Flaccid Paralysis and non-paralytic polio became renamed as meningitis. Thus in one stroke nearly all cases of polio were abolished. Today in the USA there are more cases of Acute Flaccid Paralysis, with identical clinical symptoms to paralytic polio, than there were cases of paralytic polio during the great polio epidemics.[197]

The article then went on to list six common "misconceptions" about vaccination.

CDC and Health Canada Misconception 1 is: "Diseases had already begun to disappear before vaccines were introduced, because of better hygiene and sanitation."

Craig Rebuttal: No one says diseases began to "disappear," although some, like the bubonic plague did. What they are saying is that the "death rates" dropped. Once again the CDC and Health Canada are using morbidity and mortality rates synonymously.

The article then goes on to say, "Varicella (chicken pox) can also be used to illustrate the point, since modern sanitation has obviously not prevented cases from occurring each year – with almost all children getting the disease sometime in their childhood, just as they did 20 years ago, or 80 years ago. If diseases were disappearing, we should expect varicella to be disappearing with the rest of them."

Craig Rebuttal: The point is that no one else expects diseases to "disappear." They expect them to be treated and people to be cured. Childhood diseases are necessary in order to prime immature immune systems. Surely we should have learned not to mess with Nature? Which is worse: a child with chicken pox or the adults suffering from shingles – a side-effect of varicella vaccine – that is extremely painful, more severe, and with longer side-effects?

The CDC and Health Canada's assertion under the first misconception is that developed countries that have let their vaccination levels drop have experienced epidemics. "In Sweden, the annual incidence rate of pertussis per 100,000 children 0 – 6 years of age increased from 700 cases in 1981 to 3,200 in 1985."

Craig Rebuttal: This is hardly surprising since whooping cough outbreaks tend to in three-four year cycles. Needless to say, they are using morbidity figures again and they don't quote Ström[198] who pointed out that complications after pertussis are not as high as those after vaccination.

If the CDC and Health Canada think that hygiene and sanitation are not related to infectious disease, should they be in business? It is well known that

[197] Roberts, Janine "Fear of the Invisible p63-68

[198] Ström, J. Is universal vaccination against pertussis always justified? *British Medical Journal*, October 22, 1960

overcrowding and poverty are contributing factors to a higher incidence of infectious disease. For example, the California Department of Health Services reported in 1990 that during a 27,000-case measles epidemic in the US, 45% of cases occurred in California. Of these, 10% were found in a low income rural farming area. A disproportionate number of those 352 children suffered significant complications. A further study revealed that these children came from families with a lower standard of living.

Even though 80% of infants were vaccinated against polio, an epidemic of 1031 cases occurred in Taiwan in 1982. Studies of the epidemic showed that children were five times more likely to contract paralytic polio if they received water from non-municipal rather than municipal sources.[199]

CDC and Health Canada's misconception 2:   "The majority of people getting disease have been fully immunized."

Craig Rebuttal: Are we not to accept evidence from studies in medical journals? There are numerous accounts of disease outbreaks where a high percentage of cases have been vaccinated.

The CDC and Health Canada then acknowledge that outbreaks occur in highly vaccinated populations but they explain with a hypothetical example: "In a high school of 1,000 students, none has ever had measles. All but 30 of the students have had their dose of measles vaccine, and so are considered vaccinated. However, among these 970, there would be about 97 who are not protected by the vaccine. When the student body is exposed to measles, every susceptible student becomes infected because measles is highly contagious. The 30 unvaccinated students will be infected, of course. But of the 970 who have been vaccinated, we would expect the 97 who are not protected to fall ill. Therefore, 97/127, or about 76% of the cases are fully vaccinated.

"As you can see, this doesn't prove the vaccine didn't work – only that most of the children in the class had been vaccinated, so the vaccine failures outnumbered the unvaccinated susceptibles. Looking at it another way, 100% of the children who were not vaccinated got measles compared with only 10% of those who were." (Emphasis mine.)

Craig Rebuttal: None of their statements are supported by research. To state that all unvaccinated children "will be infected of course" assumes that during an epidemic 100% of people will contract the disease. This is clearly not, nor ever has been, the case. Nor do they balance their argument with the harm done by the vaccine, perhaps because they refuse to acknowledge that vaccines have side-effects.

---

[199] Neustaedter, R. *The Vaccine Guide*. North Atlantic Books, 2002

One of the distractions with this type of argument is that we lose sight of the question about the necessity for the vaccine in the first place. *As there were only 17 deaths from measles in the whole of the USA over four years*, why was the vaccine necessary? Who made the decision to manufacture it?

CDC and Health Canada's misconception 3: Apparently vaccines are safe because "reports of adverse events are only suspicions that are temporally associated with receipt of vaccine."

Craig Rebuttal: Why are we warned about the side-effects of all prescription medicines but not of vaccines? Why do surgeons warn us of complications prior to surgery? Why are vaccines exempt from normal informed consent protocols? What drives the CDC and Health Canada to relentlessly push for vaccination?

The third misconception continues with, "While vaccines are known to cause minor, temporary side effects like soreness or fever, there is little, if any, evidence linking vaccination with permanent health problems or death."

Craig Rebuttal: Is this because evidence, such as that linking thimerosal and autism, reported in Kennedy's article, is being suppressed? Why is there a long list of health problems listed on Health Canada's Report of a Vaccine-Associated Adverse Event if these problems do not occur? Why were 38,787 adverse events reported to the US Vaccine Adverse Event Reporting System (VAERS) between 1991 and 1994?[200] Why has the Vaccine Injury Compensation Program (VICP) paid out millions of dollars in compensation despite the fact that adverse events are rarely reported?

What long-term evaluation studies, using randomized control groups, have been done to measure the results of vaccination campaigns? (The answer is none, but would they admit that fact?)

The CDC and Health Canada's misconception 4 is the same as the third: "Vaccines cause many harmful side effects, illnesses, and even death – not to mention possible long-term effects we don't even know about."

Craig Rebuttal: Like SV40 monkey virus in the polio vaccine perhaps? They then state that vaccines are very safe because they say so.

The article then goes on with the unproven assertion that, "If there were not vaccines, there would be many more cases of disease ..." What do they mean by disease? Infectious disease? We are experiencing unprecedented rates of chronic disease like asthma, autism, obesity, cancer and heart disease. As for mumps, measles and chicken pox, the statistics show that deaths from these diseases declined long before mass vaccination began despite what the CDC and Health Canada's propaganda sheet states. In addition to the statistics already quoted, here are the quinquennial average death rates of infants under one year per 1,000 live

---

[200] Null, Gary. *Vaccines: A Second Opinion.* Report on line, 2000

births in New Zealand as in the table below. These are from infectious diseases prior to vaccination.[201]

Period	Death rate	Period	Death rate	Period	Death rate
1872-1876	13.5	1902-1906	5.5	1927-1931	1.5
1877-1881	10.2	1907-1911	5.9	1932-1936	1.5
1882-1886	9.3	1912-1916	3.6	1937-1941	1.4
1887-1891	8.9	1917-1921	3.2	1942-1946	1.1
1892-1896	9.8	1922-1926	1.8	1947-1951	0.6
1897-1901	6.1				

Similar declines are shown for tuberculosis, infantile convulsions, respiratory diseases, gastric and intestinal diseases and malformations. These recorded declines in death rates are similar in other industrialised nations.

Why does the CDC and Health Canada portray vaccines as being indispensable and better at disease protection than our own immune systems, which clearly did the job before the advent of vaccines? After all, given adequate nutrition, clean water and sanitation, our innate biological defences were designed to protect us from invaders without pharmaceutical agents.

CDC and Health Canada's misconception 5: "Vaccine-preventable diseases have been virtually eliminated from the US and Canada, so there is no need for my child to be vaccinated."

Craig Rebuttal: The term "vaccine-preventable" disease suggests the unsubstantiated idea that diseases are only prevented through the use of vaccines. As the evidence does not support this assumption, this term is a subtle form of propaganda: say it often enough and people will believe it.

The CDC and Health Canada then resort to fear-mongering: the relatively few cases of disease – and they must mean infectious disease – we currently have "could very quickly become tens of thousands of cases without the protection we get from vaccines." The CDC and Health Canada need to study and honestly report the statistics of the last two centuries.

CDC and Health Canada's misconception 6: "Giving a child multiple vaccinations for different diseases at the same time increases the risk of harmful side effects and can overload the immune system." Their argument is that children

---

[201] Butler, H&P. *Just a Little Prick.* Robert Reisinger Memorial Trust, New Zealand, 2006, p.33

are continually exposed to germs in the mouth and nose and that they consume them in food.

Craig Rebuttal: The body has defence mechanisms to deal with foreign invaders through normal routes. Injecting toxins into a child's bloodstream is a quite different matter, as the body is not normally invaded that way.

Without references the CDC and Health Canada say "a number of studies have been conducted to examine the effects of giving various combinations of vaccines simultaneously." Who conducted these studies? Normally vaccine studies, when they are done at all, are performed by the pharmaceutical company who manufactures the vaccine. Who funded the studies? Where are the references? Do they suppose that no member of the general public is interested or capable of reading these studies?

If the CDC and Health Canada are to convince me that vaccinations improve health outcomes they need to replicate two studies: one conducted by the New Zealand Immunization Awareness Society in 2001 that compared the incidence of 11 chronic conditions in 226 vaccinated children with 269 unvaccinated children,[202] and another conducted by Generation Rescue in 2007 that compared the rates of autism, Attention Deficit Disorder (ADD) and other disorders in vaccinated and unvaccinated children. The results are shown below.

The New Zealand study results:

Condition	Vaccinated children with condition	% of total vaccinated children	Unvaccinated children with condition	% of total unvaccinated children
Asthma	34	15.04	8	2.97
Eczema	63	27.88	34	12.64
Glue ear	56	24.78	16	5.95
Grommets	14	6.19	2	0.74
Tonsillitis	26	11.50	3	1.12
Tonsillectomy	12	5.31	0	0.00
Apnoea	14	6.19	4	1.49
Hyperactivity	13	5.75	4	1.49
Diabetes	0	0.00	0	0.00
Epilepsy	4	1.77	0	0.00
Slow motor skill development	6	2.65	4	1.49

('Grommets' are ventilation tubes inserted into the ears of children with otitis media -- glue ear, and apnoea means periods of no breathing.) Breastfeeding was not a factor in this study as there was no significant difference in numbers of children who were breastfed or in the length of time breastfeeding continued.

---

[202] IAS. Unvaccinated children are healthier. *Waves*, Spring/Summer, 2002

Sample size in the Generation Rescue survey was 17,674 of which 991 were unvaccinated. Results showed a strong correlation between rates of neurological disorders and childhood vaccinations. Among more than 9,000 boys age 4-17, vaccinated boys were two and a half times (155%) more likely to have neurological disorders, 224% more likely to have ADD and 61% more likely to have autism than their unvaccinated peers. Older vaccinated boys, age 11-17, were 158% more likely to have a neurological disorder, 317% more likely to have ADD and 112% more likely to have autism.[203]

Why should parent groups be required to conduct studies that should be done by the CDC and government health authorities? Could it be that these authorities know that the results will be devastating to their policy of maintaining immunization rates whatever the cost?

Here is an announcement[204] from the World Health Organization, a political group composed of the health ministers of several countries:

"WHO announces push to eradicate polio: 250 million children to be immunized during 2004

International campaigns have brought polio – which used to paralyze and cripple hundreds of thousands of children every year – to the verge of elimination. But the disease has persisted in a few countries – even increased and spreading back into some areas in recent years."

Health ministers from six nations signed a declaration committing themselves to the plan, but added they will need an extra $150 million in donations beyond the money already available under the Global Polio Eradication Initiative.

The statement that polio, "used to paralyze and cripple hundreds of thousands of children every year" is not supported by data but is typical of the hyperbole used by health organizations hell bent on selling vaccines. We also have to ask why is WHO using in the Developing World the live polio vaccine no longer used in the West because it is reported to cause polio?

On May 3, 2002, the BBC News carried a headline: *Measles Vaccine's African Success Story*. The article tells us that the WHO vaccination campaign immunized 24 million children in seven countries. The number of deaths fell from 160 in 1996 to zero in 2000. What the article did not tell us is that the WHO also distributed Vitamin A – known to reduce child mortality in developing countries – and mosquito nets – known to prevent deaths from malaria.

Are WHO, FDA and CDC and Health Canada saviours of the human race with their promotion of vaccines? Or are they more concerned with wealth rather than health?

---

[203] http://www.generationrescue.org/survey.html
[204] www.msnbc.msn.com

Chapter 15

Selling a Vaccine in the 21st Century

People who watched commercial television in 2007 in North America were subjected to a barrage of advertising for a vaccine, produced by Merck, called Gardasil. A pre-pubescent girl, dressed in an indie-rocker T-shirt, scowls fiercely into the camera and says, "I want to be one less woman who will battle cervical cancer." Cut to a basement where she's pounding drums. She nonchalantly twirls a drumstick. "One less," she asserts as though defying argument.

Other commercials show 'cool' girls engaging in wholesome, but unlikely, activities. One is having her hand taped in preparation for a boxing bout with a punch bag. Another skateboards with dreadlocks flying. One says, "Each year in the US thousands of women learn they have cervical cancer. I could be one less."

A mother appears with bad news: "Gardasil may not protect everyone," she says tenderly and then lists the side effects: pain, swelling, itching, redness at injection site, nausea. She doesn't mention death or paralysis.

Having a mother voice the downside of Gardasil is the equivalent of a parent explaining the dangers of smoking – virtually a guarantee that the teen will assert her independence and get herself vaccinated.

Gardasil is a vaccine intended to protect women against two strains of the human papilloma virus (HPV) that reportedly is linked to cervical cancer. It was approved by the FDA (Food and Drug Administration) in June 2006 and then recommended by the CDC (Centers for Disease Control) for females ages 9 to 26. The series of three shots costs $360, making it the most expensive vaccine on record. The major problem underlying the Gardasil campaign is that HPV does not cause cervical cancer.

Two statements by the FDA are listed on its website.[205]: The first is "*most infections (by HPV) are short-lived and not associated with cervical cancer.*"

A second is a news release of March 31, 2003 that states,[206] "The HPV DNA test is not intended to substitute for regular Pap screening. Nor is it intended to

---

[205] http://www.fda.gov/ohrms/dockets/dockets/07p0210/07p-0210-ccp0001-01-vol1.pdf
[206] http://www.fda.gov/bbs/topics/NEWS/2003/NEW00890.html

screen women under 30 who have normal Pap tests. Although the rate of HPV infection in this group is high, most infections are short-lived and **not associated with cervical cancer**." (Emphasis added.)

Furthermore, the FDA states in the same press release, "*Most women who become infected with HPV are able to eradicate the virus and suffer no apparent long-term consequences to their health.*"

If the FDA knew in 2003 that most HPV infections are not associated with cervical cancer and that HPV infections resolve themselves, why did it approve a vaccine in June 2006?

If you are looking for a sound financial investment, then Merck is your best bet. Jim Cramer, on TV's *Wall Street Confidential*, said in November, 2007, "... (the) vaccine from Merck is going to be huge. It's going from about $300 million to $4 billion in revenue over the next year, and that's just one vaccine."

Cramer went on to explain, "For years, vaccines were risky, because if something went wrong, it was only a matter of time before a company had a class-action suit against it. So the drug companies pretty much decided there was no real money in vaccines. One of the big changes the analysts didn't pick up on is that since then, the plaintiff's bar has been beaten back, so the litigation risk of vaccines has declined."

The raising of the plaintiff's bar refers to the protection of vaccine manufacturers conferred by the National Vaccine Injury Compensation Act (NVICA). The NVICA, a "no-fault" compensation system, was passed in 1986 to shield the pharmaceutical industry from civil litigation due to problems associated with vaccines. Under the law, families of vaccine-injured persons are required to file a petition which may be heard by a Special Master in the vaccine court. Successful claims are paid from a Trust Fund that is managed by the Department of Health and Human Services, with Justice Department attorneys acting as the legal representatives of the Fund. Processing a claim through the vaccine court can take up to 10 years and it is estimated that less than 25% of those who qualify for a hearing actually receive compensation.

In other words, Cramer is telling us that now people can't sue for damages from a pharmaceutical product, it is okay to make a vaccine, regardless of whether it is needed or effective, and there is no need to worry about it being harmful.

Lost in all the Gardasil advertising hype are a few facts:

* The majority of women clear the HPV virus from their bodies naturally but women with risk factors, such as smoking, long-time use of oral contraceptives, and co-infection with herpes simplex virus or chlamydia, are at higher risk for chronic HPV infection.
* Between 1955 and 1992, cervical cancer deaths in American women dropped by 74 percent due to routine pap smears.

* There are about 9,800 new cases of cervical cancer annually diagnosed in the U.S., which represents .007 percent out of the approximately 1,372,000 new cancer cases of all types diagnosed.
* There are about 3,700 deaths in mostly older American women annually attributed to HPV- related cervical cancer, which is about .006 percent of the approximately 570,000 cancer deaths that occur in the U.S.
* Most cervical pre-cancers develop slowly, so nearly all cervical cancers can be prevented with regular pap smear screening and prompt treatment.[207]

We live with viruses – millions of them. HPV swims in a sea of viruses that, in people with a functioning immune system, do not cause a problem. In those women with a compromised immune system, HPV is a tell-tale sign of cervical cancer even though it is not the cause. They are like cops who show up at an accident – they are present but did not cause the accident.

Nevertheless, in 2007 a number of States added Gardasil to the list of mandatory vaccinations for entering school although, after public outcry, a few have thought better of it.[208]

According to Merck, Gardasil, in clinical trials, was shown to be 100% effective in preventing infection with HPV strains 16 and 18, which it says cause about 70% of cervical cancer cases. How would they know if something prevented something? Cervical cancer typically develops in mid-life even though HPV exposure typically occurs at sexual debut. Therefore, the vaccine is purported to protect against a disease that may occur, or may not, about 30-35 years after HPV infection. Yet the duration of the "protection" given by the vaccine is unknown.

According to the National Vaccine Information Center "the FDA allowed Merck to use a potentially reactive aluminium-containing placebo as a control for most trial participants, rather than a non-reactive saline solution placebo."[209] Using a reactive placebo can artificially increase the appearance of safety of an experimental drug or vaccine in a clinical trial. Gardasil contains 225 mcg of aluminium and, although aluminium adjuvants have been used in vaccines for decades, they were never tested for safety in clinical trials. Merck and the FDA did not disclose how much aluminium was in the placebo.

Aluminium is a heavy metal with known neurotoxic effects on human and animal nervous systems. In 1996, the American Academy of Pediatrics issued a position paper on Aluminium Toxicity in Infants and Children which stated in the first paragraph, "Aluminum is now being implicated as interfering with a variety of cellular and metabolic processes in the nervous system and in other tissues.[210]

---

[207] National Vaccine Information Centre, *One Less? Evaluating the High Cost of Gardasil*, December 17, 2007
[208] http://www.ncsl.org/programs/health/HPVvaccine.htm#hpvlegis
[209] www.909shot.com
[210] http://www.whale.to/vaccine/palevsky.html

A review of the medical literature on aluminium reveals a surprising lack of scientific evidence that injected aluminium is safe. There is limited understanding of what happens to children when aluminium is injected into their bodies, including whether or not it accumulates in tissues and organs or is properly eliminated from the body. It is also unknown if genetic factors affect long term adverse health outcomes for those injected with aluminium-containing vaccines.

Nearly 90% of all Gardasil recipients and 85% of those who received the "placebo" reported one or more adverse events within 15 days of vaccination. Pain and swelling at the site of injection affected approximately 83% of Gardasil recipients and 73% of those who received the aluminium placebo. About 60% of those who received either the vaccine or the placebo had systemic adverse events including headache, fever, nausea, dizziness, vomiting, diarrhoea and myalgia. Those who received the vaccine reported even more serious adverse events such as gastroenteritis, appendicitis, pelvic inflammatory disease, asthma, bronchospasm and arthritis.

With regards to long-term safety, one sentence in the vaccine's insert is particularly revealing. "Gardasil has not been evaluated for the potential to cause carcinogenicity or genotoxicity." Carcinogenicity means the ability to cause cancer and genotoxicity means chromosome damage.

No drug is without side effects and those of vaccines, as we have seen, can be devastating. Between June 2006, when Gardasil was approved, and October 2007, more than 4,000 Gardasil adverse events had been reported to the Vaccine Adverse Events Reporting System. (VAERS).[211] Although approximately 75% of these were those listed by the mother in the ad, there were also:

- More than 40 cases of Guillain-Barré syndrome
- 11 deaths including one 12-year old
- 28 pregnant women who miscarried.

That was for the first 14 months. By 2009, in the US alone, over 10,000 adverse reactions, including 29 deaths, had been reported to the Vaccine Adverse Event Reporting System.

Gardasil contains thimerosal; the long-term effects of injecting mercury into the bloodstream of girls who already have received other mercury-laced vaccines is unknown.

Research published in the *Journal of the American Medical Association* (August, 2007),[212] entitled, "Effect of Human Papillomavirus 16/18 L1 Viruslike Particle Vaccine Among Young Women With Pre-existing Infection" by Hildesheim et al. makes interesting reading. The study sought to determine the

---

[211] www.medalerts.org/vaersdb/index.html
[212] http://jama.ama-assn.org/cgi/content/full/298/7/743/DC1

usefulness of the HPV vaccine among women who already carry HPV (which includes virtually all women who are sexually active, regardless of their age).

The conclusion of the study reads: *"In women positive for HPV DNA, HPV-16/18 vaccination does not accelerate clearance of the virus and should not be used to treat prevalent infections."*

The body of the text includes: ***"No significant evidence of a vaccine therapeutic effect was observed in analyses restricted to women who received all doses of vaccine or those with evidence of single HPV infections at entry... "***

In other words, the authors found no evidence that the vaccine worked at all in HPV infected women. Furthermore the authors state: *"... rates of viral clearance over a 12-month period are not influenced by vaccination."* Which means that the vaccine did not destroy the viruses within a year. If it didn't affect existing viruses, how can it prevent their appearance in girls when they become sexually active?

The article goes on to make statements that should cause every doctor and health authority around the world to rethink Gardasil vaccination policies: *"Results from our community-based study provide strong evidence that there is little, if any, therapeutic benefit from the vaccine in the population we studied. Furthermore, we see no reason to believe that there is therapeutic benefit of the vaccine elsewhere because the biological effect of vaccination among already infected women is not expected to vary by population."*

What baffles me about this Gardasil campaign is the gullibility of the American public. Very few people seem to possess working crap-detectors and those few who do are subject to abuse if they dare to voice criticism of vaccines. Any discussion about vaccination quickly becomes hostile. For example, in a *New York Times* debate following an article on March 21, 2008, about the connection between vaccines and autism, individuals wrote the following:

"I'm so tired of these morons who refuse to vaccinate their children. It's stupid and selfish and, as usual, the kid suffers because of an hysterical, paranoid mother. What we need is a vaccine against paranoid conspiracy theory nuts. Oh, yeah....and by all means, let's trust a primary care doc from Arizona rather than the AAP and CDC. After all, what does some pinhead in private practice know that the best trained, most informed academic docs at some backwater like Johns Hopkins or CHOP or Children's Boston know, anyhow."

The AAP is the American Academy of Pediatricians which strongly endorses government vaccination policies. The AAP is known to have clear conflicts of interest with the vaccine manufacturers. For instance, private letters documenting significant contributions made by vaccine manufacturers to them are on record.[213]

"The irrational decisions of adults, including parents and even physicians, supported by superstition, faith and magical beliefs, rather than data, evidence and proof, cannot stand in the way of science's obligation to create new knowledge to protect the members of a society, especially its most vulnerable members."

---

[213] http://www.ageofautism.com/2008/01/aap-its-time-fo.html

"The parents whose personal beliefs cause them to fail to vaccinate their children should be seen clearly for what they are - child abusers. They are as monstrous as people that allow their children to die because they are convinced that if their god wants their children to live, he'll take care of it."

Even doctors weighed in:

"As an epidemiologist who believes in the power and strength of herd immunity, I would like to ask these people who forgo vaccination to politely leave the herd."

To me this statement demonstrates the power and strength of herd mentality.

"They (unvaccinated children) *should not be permitted in clinics and hospitals, where immunocompromised children and adults have the right to safety. No exception, whether based on religious faith or just garden-variety ignorance and superstition."*

Why this desperate need to defend a belief in vaccines? Would the same rage be expressed if the debate was over insulin or an anti-hypertensive drug? We do not seem to have progressed as a human species since Bruno was burnt at the stake for upholding Copernicus's conviction that the sun, not the earth, was the centre of the solar system.

Chapter 16

Sacred Cows

(Definition: Medical procedures unreasonably immune to criticism.)

I made a Victoria sponge and a pot of Yorkshire tea in preparation for another visit from D. I had sent her the chapter on Influenza to ask if she minded my using her name and then she wanted to see all I had written.

"I take it you don't believe in vaccination," D said after we settled down.

"It's not a question of *belief*, D. This isn't a religion that rests on faith. Though sometimes, I have to wonder. A recent NVIC newsletter told me that Professor John Oxford, Britain's leading flu expert, said the development of a universal vaccine was the "holy grail" of flu research. Holy grail? Do they want us to believe that their creations are holy?"

"Aren't they?" D said.

"I find it interesting that when I say I am writing about vaccination some people promptly go into defence mode and mutter about controversy. Would they react in the same way if I said I was writing about prophylactic antibiotics in cows? Or about hernia supports?"

D laughed. "Are you? Writing about hernia supports, I mean?"

I hurrumphed. "Western medicine is supposed to be scientific. The catch phrase in medicine and nursing is 'evidence-based.' So the question to ask of vaccination is, 'what is the evidence that it prevents disease?'"

"What about health authorities' evidence?"

"That's what I've examined. I have found none that shows that any vaccine prevents any disease but I found plenty of evidence of harm."

"Surely they must do some good?"

"No. They simply damage the immune system. Look, D, if vaccination prevented disease, why do the vaccinated get the disease when there's an outbreak of it? A true scientist posits a theory and then sets out to disprove the theory. Statistical hypotheses are worded to disprove, not prove. So if you theorise that your vaccine will prevent fulminating foot rot, you give it to 95% of the population and in the next outbreak, 65% of the vaccinated get it, what does that say about your theory?"

"Not a whole lot," D said. "But I don't understand why doctors and nurses go on with it."

"They are caught between an intellectual rock and a corporate hard place. People have an astounding ability to believe what they want to believe in order to make it appear reasonable and logical." I picked up my notebook and thumbed through it. "George Bernard Shaw said, 'Faith may be manufactured in any degree of magnitude and intensity – not only without any basis of fact or reason, but in open contradiction of both – simply by a *fervent desire* to believe, coupled by *a personal interest in believing.*' And doctors and nurses sure have a personal interest in believing. This human weakness has caused health authorities to ignore clear signals of the dangers of vaccination to the point where I wonder about their ethics."

"What's that?" D pointed to the notebook.

"It's notes I've made of quotations I wanted to use." I flicked through the pages. "Here's one I never found a place for; quoted in *Wake Up to Health.*[214] Dr. Peter Marsh said of SARS, 'The fact is that 260 people have died. But for every Chinese person who has died, 10 million have not. In an ordinary rational world, that sounds like quite good odds, but not in this context. In this country (UK), every year 1500 people are killed falling down the stairs. The implication would be that people should only be allowed to build bungalows.' Would that such common sense be more common!"

"What prevents the medical community from accepting the evidence of harm from vaccinations?"

"I guess they are comfortable with their received knowledge. They can't be expected to go back to the roots of it all. But when they do find out that that knowledge is false, what I can't understand is the emotional reaction. I've been reading the Dalai Lama's *The Universe in a Single Atom.* There's one passage I love: "To deny the authority of empirical evidence is to disqualify oneself as someone worthy of critical engagement in a dialogue." Isn't that wonderful? *Worthy of critical engagement in a dialogue.* How many health professionals are worthy? His Holiness did not say if others may disqualify people, but there's a lot of health professionals I would disqualify."

"You talk about the myth of vaccination; is it a myth?"

"When a version of events is repeated so often that it becomes accepted as fact by the majority of people, even when there is no supporting evidence, then a myth is born. And myths are very difficult to shift. As that wise 19th century physician, Hadwen said, in *Truth* in 1923, 'When once an error is accepted by a profession corporately and endowed by government, to uproot it becomes a Herculean task, beside which the entrance of a rich man into the Kingdom of

---

[214] Ransom, S. *Wake Up To Health.* Credence Publications, 2003

Heaven is easy.' Plenty of people have attempted this Herculean task," I said as I waved at my basket of books on vaccination. "The information is there for anyone who cares to find it."

D began to forage in the basket. "The authors are certainly well qualified," she said. "Most have Ph.Ds. What's OMD?"

"That must be Neustaedter; he's a doctor of Oriental medicine. His is a very good book for parents. Here's one written by a chiropractor, Tim O'Shea. I've gone over these books so much I feel as if I know the authors personally."

"I'm looking for a reference for my daughter. What do you suggest?"

"Does she want Vaccination 100, 200 or 300?" I said.

"What do you mean?"

"Some, like Miller, are written for parents; others like Null's report and Scheibner's book are reviews of the medical literature and take some time and concentration to read. Actually, Miller's latest book, *Vaccine Safety Manual*, is a must-read."[215]

"I'll ask her. Where did you get all these articles?" D opened the bin of files of articles.

"From the internet. Some people sneer at the internet as an information source but it depends on what the source is, not on how the information is transferred. Using the net you can get into the National Library of Medicine in Washington for medical and nursing journals. I've used *The Lancet* and *British Medical Journal* sites quite a lot and there is a wonderful site for historical stuff called Whale. Then you can get the *Congressional Records* and quite a few newspapers and magazines."

"Here's a book written by an MD. Should I suggest this to my daughter?"

"Why is a book written by an MD more valid than one written by a Ph.D? After all, a Ph.D is a higher degree than an MD."

"I dunno." D laughed. "I expect they know something about medicine."

"So do some Ph.Ds. But what a Ph.D can do is interpret research studies and analyse and synthesise data; no matter what the topic."

"This one by Cave and Michell, *What Your Doctor May Not Tell You About Children's Vaccinations*," D said, holding up the book. "What's it like?"

"It's good for explaining side-effects but on page 10 they say, 'A more scientific approach was used in the late eighteenth century when Edward Jenner, who discovered that inoculating people with the animal disease cowpox made people immune to the deadly human disease smallpox. This was an interesting concept, and fortunately for Jenner it helped save lives, but the use of an animal disease to treat humans also presented the possibility that other diseases could be introduced along with the intended virus.' Quite clearly they have not done their homework. I cannot understand why people who should know better continue to assert that putting cowpox pus under people's skin saved them from smallpox. The figures say otherwise. And to call it a scientific approach! Does no one wonder

---

[215] Miller, N.Z. *Vaccine Safety Manual*. New Atlantean Press, 2008

about the effects of passing viruses back and forth between animals and humans? Words fail me."

"I wish they would," D said unkindly.

I ignored the hint. "Then on page 18 they say, 'We are fortunate that we have stopped the epidemics of smallpox, polio, diphtheria and measles. The introduction of vaccines has accomplished more than we dreamed they would.' They sure have; we now have unprecedented epidemics of diabetes, autism, neurological disorders, asthma, attention deficit disorder – you name it. You have only to look at the death rates for childhood diseases before and after the introduction of vaccination to know that vaccines had no effect. Dr. Cave is perpetuating the myth and because she is an MD people will believe her."

D ruffled through the book. "They do tell US parents how to get exemptions." She looked up. "I can hardly believe that the Land of the Free forces its citizens to have vaccinations."

"Bizarre isn't it? If they are so beneficial people would line up for them. And you would think that the most vaccinated children in the world would be the healthiest. They are not. It's shameful that the US is 34th on the list of infant mortality rates in the world. What you commonly see now is, not only kids with metal in their mouths, but fatsoes with inhalers. But that's OK as long as they don't get measles."

D raised her eyebrows. "If vaccination was stopped, wouldn't there be huge epidemics of disease?"

"I assume you mean infectious disease? Death rates had declined before vaccination started and that's what really matters. Experiencing infectious disease has been part of the human condition since man has walked the earth. Why do the vaccarazo insist on assuming that a healthy immune system is incapable of dealing with that experience? Or benefiting from it? Where is the evidence that it is good to never, ever get measles? Or chicken pox? Or that "universal" vaccines will not put pressure on microorganisms to mutate into vaccine-resistant strains?"

"Do you think your book will stop vaccination?"

"No, of course not. A huge and extraordinarily lucrative industry has been built up around it. If I can make a few people, particularly parents, think, and if I can save them the agony of watching their healthy babies turn into a zombies, then I'll be satisfied. But the important thing for me is that I have spoken my truth. That's all I can do."

"How would you summarize your research on vaccination?" D asked as she stacked the cups and saucers.

"Vaccination is the biggest medical scam of the twentieth century with iatrogenic consequences that will take decades to mop up."

THE END

Bibliography

Allen, A. *Vaccine. The Controversial Story of Medicine's Greatest Lifesaver.* W.W. Norton & Company, 2007

Barry, I. *Portrait of Lady Mary Wortley Montagu.* Ernest Menn Ltd. 1928

Butler H & P, *Just a Little Prick.* Robert Reisinger Memorial Trust, New Zealand, 2006

Butler H & P, *From One Prick to Another.* Robert Reisinger Memorial Trust, New Zealand, 2008

Carrol, Lewis. *The Annotated Alice* with notes by Martin Gardner. Bramhall House, 1960

Cave, S. & Mitchell, D. *What Your Doctor May Not Tell You About Children's Vaccinations.* Warner Books, 2001

Chaitow, L. *Vaccination and Immunization: Dangers, Delusions, Alternatives.* C.W. Daniel Company Limited, 1987

Cornoyer, C. *What About Immunizations? A Parents Guide to Informed Decision-making.* Private Research Publication, Canby, Oregon, 1987

Coulter, HL & Fisher, BL. *A Shot in the Dark.* Avery Publishing Group Inc. 1991

Creighton, C. *Jenner and Vaccination: a Strange Chapter of Medical History.* Swan Sonnerschein & Co. 1889.

Day, P. *Health Wars.* Credence Publications, 2001

Duesberg, PH. *Inventing the AIDS Virus.* Regnery Publishing, 1996

Ellison, S. *Health Myths Exposed.* Authorhouse, 2004

Evans, RG, Barer, ML, Marmor, TR. *Why Are Some People Healthy and Others Not?* Aldine de Gruyter, New York, 1994

Golden, I. *Vaccination? A Review of Risks and Alternatives.* Australia, 1994

Haggard, H. *Devils, Drugs and Doctors.* Harper, 1929. Pocket Book Edition 1946

Hale, AR. *The Medical Voodoo.* Gotham House Inc. 1935

Halsband, R. *The Life of Lady Mary Wortley Montagu.* Clarendon Press, 1956

Halvorsen, R. *The Truth About Vaccines.* Gibson Square, 2007

Hume, D. *Bechamp or Pasteur: a Lost Chapter in the History of Biology.* Kessinger Publishing,1922

James, W. *Immunizations: The Reality Beyond the Myth.* Bergin & Gervey, 1988

Johnson. S. *The Ghost Map.* Riverhead Books, 2006

Kalokerinos, A. *Every Second Child.* Nelson, Ltd. Australia. 1974

Kirby, D. *Evidence of Harm.* St. Martin's Press, New York, 2005

Lanctot, G. *The Medical Mafia.* Quebec, 1995

Lydall, W. *Raising a Vaccine Free Child.* AuthorHouse, 2005

McBean, E. *The Poisoned Needle.* Health Research, Pomeroy. WA, 1993

Mendelsohn, R. *How to Raise a Healthy Child in Spite of your Doctor*, Random House, 1987

Miller, N. *Immunization: Theory vs. Reality.* New Atlantean Press, 1995

Miller, N.Z. *Vaccines: Are They Really Safe and Effective?* New Atlantean Press, New Mexico, 1992
Miller, NZ. *Vaccine Safety Manual.* New Atlantean Press, New Mexico, 2008
Neustaedter, R. *The Vaccine Guide.* North Atlantic Books, 2002
O'Shea, T. *The Sanctity of Human Blood: Vaccination IS not Immunization.* Two Trees, San Jose, California, 2004
Oshinsky, DM. *Polio: An American Story.* Oxford University Press, 2005
Ransom, S. *Wake Up to Health in the Twenty First Century.* Credence Publications, 2003
Roberts, J. *Fear of the Invisible.* Impact Investigative Media Productions, 2008, Second Edition 2009.
Scheibner, V. *Vaccination: 100 Years of Orthodox Research Shows that Vaccination Represents a Medical Assault on the Immune System.* New Atlantean Press, 1993
Scheibner, V. *Behavioural Problems in Childhood: the Link to Vaccination.* Griffin Press, 2002
Sinclair, I. *Vaccination: The "Hidden" Facts.* Australia, 1992
Swan, J. *The Vaccination Problem.* 1936, www.whale.to
Tobyn, G. *Culpeppers' Medicine.* Element Books Ltd. 1997

ARTICLES

Alderson, M. International Mortality Statistics. *Facts on File*, Inc. 1981
Ayoub, D. Thimerosol: Definite cause of autism. *Scoop*, March 2005
Bayly, MB. The Story of the Salk Anti-Poliomyelitis Vaccine. www.whale.to
Bernard, S. et al. Autism: a novel form of mercury poisoning. www.mercola.com
Bird, C. To Be Or Not To Be? 150 Years of Hidden Knowledge. *Nexus* magazine, April 1992
Byers, RK & Moll, FC. Encephalopathies following prophylactic pertussis vaccination. *Paediatrics.* 1(4):437-56
Carter, H. "Measles outbreak in Fife: which MMR policy." *Public Health*, January 1993
Creighton, C. Vaccination. *Encyclopaedia Britannica*, Ninth Edition, 1875-1889, www.whale.to
Doshi, P. Viral Marketing: The selling of the flu vaccine. *Harper's Magazine*, March 2006. Vol. 312, No. 1870
Fisher, BL. The Vaccine Reaction. Special Report of the National Vaccine Information Center, Spring 2004
Gaublomme K. Has smallpox really disappeared from the earth? www.whale.to
Givner, C. & Goldman, GS. Injection. *Medical Veritas International Inc.* 2006
Hadwen, W. The Fraud of Vaccination. *Truth,* January 3, 1923

Health! Canada Magazine, March 2001

Henderson et al. Smallpox as a biological weapon: medical and public health management. *Journal of the American Medical Association*, June 9, 1999, Vol. 281 p.3132

IAS. Unvaccinated children are healthier. *Waves*, Spring/Summer, 2002

Incao, PF. Vaccination from a Clinician's Perspective. *Well Beings*, November 1988

Jefferson, T. Influenza vaccination: policy versus evidence. *British Medical Journal*, October 28, 2006

Jenner, E. An Inquiry into the Causes and Effects of the Variolae Vaccine. 1798. www.whale.to

Jenner, E. Further Observations on the Variolae Vaccina, of Cow-pox. www.whale.to

Kennedy, RF. Deadly Immunity. *Rolling Stone,* June 20, 2005, www.whale.to

Kent, C. The Polio Vaccine Myth. *The Chiropractic Journal*, March 2000

Krasner, G. The Dangers of Vaccination. www.naturodoc.com

Mendelsohn, R. The Medical Time Bomb of Immunization Against Disease. www.whale.to

Mercola, J. Missing the Flu Diagnosis in Kids Just Another Excuse for a Vaccine. www.mercola.com

Miller, NZ. Annual Flu Deaths: The Big Lie. www.thinktwice.com

Null, G. Vaccines: a Second Opinion. www.garynull.com

O'Shea, T. Autism and mercury: the San Diego Conference. www.thedoctorwithin.com

O'Shea, T. Avian Flu: the Pandemic That Will Never Be. www.thedoctorwithin.com

O'Shea, T. The Doors of Perception: Why Americans will Believe Almost Anything. www.thedoctorwithin.com

Obomsawin, R. Immunization: a Report for CIDA, May ,1992

Obomsawin, R. Universal Immunization: Medical Miracle or Masterful Mirage. www.whale.to

Quak, T. Vaccinations and their side effects. Translated by Christian Kurz. www.lyghtforce.com/HomeopathyOnline/issue2

Ransom, S. Lies, Damn Lies and Statistics. www.campaignfortruth.com

Rattigan, P. Assault on the Species, Truth Campaign Magazine, 15

Scheibner, V. Shaken Baby Syndrome – the vaccination link. *Nexus* Magazine, Aug/Sept, 1998

Singh, VK, Sheren, XL, Yang, VC. Serological association of measles virus and human herpesvirus-6 with brain autoantibodies in autism. *Clinical Immunology and Immunopathology,* 1998; 89(1);105-8

Snicer, A. Near disaster with the Salk vaccine. *Science Digest*, December, 1963

Ström, J. Is universal vaccination against pertussis always justified? *British Medical Journal,* October 22, 1960

In Memorium

Ian.
Born June 25, 2007, died August 10, 2007. Lived for 47 days.

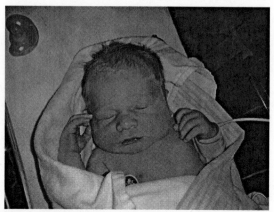

Newborn picture

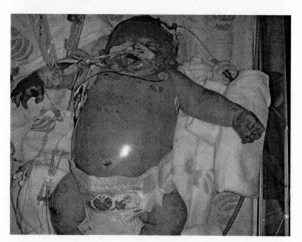

Nine days after Hepatitis B shot.

Ian – and the millions of vaccine-damaged children –
forgive us for we know not what we do.

INDEX

85, 95-102, 109,
117, 118, 121,
125, 129
VZV, 50, 51

Wakefield, Mr.
 Andrew, 70-71
Warrington, 35
Wilder, Dr. A., 13

World Health
 Organisation, 38,
 68, 84, 85, 87, 89,
 100, 101, 108,
 110, 116